AMERICAN TRIAGE

From 9/11 to *Fahrenheit 451*

AMERICAN TRIAGE
From 9/11 to *Fahrenheit 451*

Adam Axler

Introduction by
S. Thompson, MD

American Triage: From 9/11 to Fahrenheit 451 by Adam Axler.

For privacy reasons, some names, locations, and dates may have been changed.

Published in the United States and Canada by Whisk(e)y Tit: www.whiskeytit.com. If you wish to use or reproduce all or part of this book for any means, please let the author and publisher know. You're pretty much required to, legally.

Cover art and interior drawing Nancy Grossman (b.1940), *Male Figure Bound at Elbows with Head Turned Right Yet To Be Titled*, 1963, ink on paper, 16 3/4 x 13 7/8 inches / 42.5 x 35.2 cm, signed; Collection of halley k harrisburg and Michael Rosenfeld, New York; © Nancy Grossman, Courtesy of Michael Rosenfeld Gallery LLC, New York, NY

Author photo courtesy of Dreamlight Studios
Cover Design and Layout by David McNamara / Publish Publish

ISBN: 978-1-952600-68-5

Library of Congress Control Number: 2026938680

FIRST WHISKEY TIT PAPERBACK EDITION

THIS BOOK IS FOR

Lori, Sammi, and Sydney,

WHO GIVE ME ALL THAT I NEED.

THANK YOU, MY LOVES.

I WILL ALWAYS TAKE CARE OF YOU.

It's creeping in sweetly
It's definitely here
There's nothing more deadly
Than slow growing fear

—Phoebe Killdeer

"The burnout rate in Emergency Medicine is *100%*."

—Me

Triage Order

Introduction

I think it is a true saying that life is about the journey and not so much the destination. As such, what makes the journey easier at times are our companions along the way. And some of the people we meet along the road make a mark, and might even serve to enrich our lives.

Adam Axler is one of those people.

We met roughly seventeen years ago. I had recently sold my own urgent care center, and had started working at an urgent care where Adam was already employed. In retrospect, we likely worked so well together because we both had a direct, no-nonsense approach to medicine. That having been said, our major differences lay in our personality types in terms of patient interaction. Adam would say the quiet part out loud, while most of the time I would use a subtler approach. I might choose to cajole a patient, come at them sideways, whereas Adam was more straightforward.

I think then and now, as with many healthcare providers today, frustration comes from the realization that we are no longer practicing medicine that is based on good science and solid research. Medicine, to its detriment, has now fully become a *business*. We are now "providers," instead of physicians, physician assistants, and nurse practitioners. And we no longer have patients. Instead, we have "customers," essentially consumers. Our employers' evaluation of us is now based on surveys and patient impact scores. The overall push now is to find a way to say yes, and to keep the customer happy.

As to my background, I am a medical doctor, residency trained and board certified in both Emergency Medicine and Urgent Care Medicine. With disbelief, I realize that I have now been a physician going on thirty years, and thus far, I have seen a remarkable change in medicine over the years. *American Triage: From 9/11 to Fahrenheit 451* gives insight to this change through many recollections and stories from Adam's career in healthcare. He takes us from his time in Emergency Medical Services (EMS) in New York during 9/11 to his time practicing as a Physician Assistant (PA) in emergency room and urgent care settings.

What Adam explores in this memoir is the steady decline of real medicine in this country. Patients now do their own research, perhaps with Dr. Google or, now, AI, before coming to an urgent care center, and come in many times with preformed opinions as to their diagnosis and what they want for treatment. Many times, these preconceived notions are based on false information from ill-qualified sources, such as public personas, or poorly done and now-refuted research studies.

The measles outbreak that is presently worsening by the day makes this writing even more relevant to the current practice of medicine. The difficulty for trained, qualified, experienced healthcare providers now lies in trying to explain the real science of what is going on, and to somehow convince the patient of what is the proper and best treatment. Inevitably on any given day, a number of patients will politely, or not so politely inform the provider that essentially, they want what they want.

Adam's recollections from his career give insight to the current practice of urgent care, a behind-the-scenes look. He takes one through a typical day, and shows what a shift is like in this setting. On any given day there will be funny occurrences, pleasant experiences, and frustrating ones. Oftentimes frustration comes from the fact that Adam *still cares*. And he cares about practicing good medicine.

This brief memoir takes us from prehospital to emergency department and urgent care settings. The book is for everyone, from all walks of life, but particularly those that frequent these settings. Healthcare providers will likely commiserate in recognition of the nature of some of these stories. The presentation is raw, no holds barred, but also honest and amusing. With the acknowledgement that practicing good medicine is becoming at times difficult, we should ponder the potential solutions to this brewing problem before it is too late.

—S. Thompson, MD

Order Up

I can still smell the stink.

Not the stink of cat piss or roach shit in an unkempt New York City apartment. The stink of drunks doused in their own vomit and urine. The stench and menace of being punched in the face while protecting my two-year-old Down syndrome patient. Of three-day-old dead bodies and three-hour-old GI bleeds that reek of impending death. The smell of comatose ODs lying on scattered street corners. Picking them up, dropping them off, picking them up, dropping them off without one thank you.

I have ridden in pee-soaked elevators in Yonkers and the Bronx, sat twelve inches away from the bat-shittiest crazies from Randall's Island for twenty-minute rides over the bridge. I've had people give me the finger, call me every possible name while I'm coming to help them and their families.

And I will carry around that stench with me for the rest of my life.

I didn't grow up with a doctor's kit in my toy box. Nobody in my family practiced medicine and I never thought I would end up where I am today. When most of my patients saw me walk into the room they initially questioned my qualifications because, despite salt-and-pepper patches, I looked younger than I was. What they didn't see was a man who had given his entire adult life to medicine, and who was both fighting against and contributing to its destruction.

What they didn't see was a guy who worked as a paramedic at Ground Zero, who saw the falling victims and was hit with debris from the collapsing towers. Whose wife was on a plane from LaGuardia to Pittsburgh that morning . . . They didn't see a guy who had shocked a man back to life on a crowded New York City street corner in front of hundreds of people, intubated him on the ground, and had him breathing and conscious five minutes later. And they didn't see a man who received medals from the city of New York for pulling elderly patients out of a burning building.

They didn't see a guy who had found people hanging from rafters or even from a closet rod, rotten and rigored. They didn't see a guy who had absorbed eighteen-year-olds splattered on the concrete after jumping twenty stories, or the remnants of a body run over by a subway train. Ever had to tell the parents of a six-month-old that their child is dead? I did. Ever had to tell an eighty-five-year-old woman that her husband of sixty years is dead? I've done that too.

I have taken care of stabbing victims in Times Square and gunshot wounds in Central Park. I have put back dislocated knees, shoulders, hips, elbows, toes, and fingers. I have removed BBs, dildos, tampons, cockroaches, pencil erasers, beads, carrots, and used condoms from every orifice. I have removed needles from overdosed heroin addicts. And I have diagnosed patients with leukemia, lymphoma, pancreatic cancer, colon cancer, and lung cancer both by acumen and pure luck. So, in total, I am one of a handful of people walking this earth to ever have done all of those things.

I have been given flowers, gift cards, cakes, cookies, homemade drawings, checks left for me in envelopes, money slipped into my pocket, even bibles. I have had hundreds of patients ask me to be their private doctor, hundreds of thank-you notes and personalized letters detailing the gratitude of the people I have helped. I had a group of patients who followed me from practice to practice that treated me as their regular doctor.

My coworkers entrusted me with their health and the health of their spouses and children on a regular basis. When my wife had a fever or my kids were wheezing in the middle of the night we didn't have to pick up the phone. I knew how to take care of them and the peace of mind I gave my wife was special. In those moments, I felt honored and grateful to have chosen the right profession. Unfortunately, those moments were few and far between.

What stinks though, *what really stinks?*

Summa cum laude graduate, highest honors in PA school while managing three moves, a wife, and a newborn? No, nobody gives a shit about that. Once they saw a friendly face, they treated me as if I had a Burger King crown on my head or was wearing a shirt embroidered with the Golden Arches. *Whip out your pen and paper, boy, and take this down. I need a Z-Pak and codeine cough medicine to go with those fries.*

This thing called medicine? It's no longer science, no longer deduction, no longer pieces of a puzzle. It's fucking customer service. I'm a well-trained waiter who makes sure that your wine matches your entrée, or in this case, that your antibiotic doesn't interfere with your psych meds.

You've killed it for me. Our system has devolved from

a scientific endeavor to low-level customer satisfaction. There is even a cottage industry of doctors who write books about how terrible other doctors are (and we hate you by the way).

On a weekly basis, our patients threaten to sue us if we don't give them exactly what they want, and promise us this will be the last time they will ever come to our offices. And on a weekly basis, we see those same patients again and again. The patients who decided they wanted to dictate the terms of their care and the doctors who thought it might be good to let them do so forgot one thing. *Those of us who still have to practice fucking hate it.*

I went from driving an hour each way to the ER with a naive enthusiasm that I'd be saving lives for the next twelve hours, to a four-minute urgent care commute hoping my neighbors wouldn't show up with post-divorce STDs. The fall from *I can help everyone,* to *I can still help those who need it,* to *what can I do to not get sued today?* Defensive medicine thinly veiled as "best practices."

Fifty-five-year-olds asking for speed, while also telling me medications like Seroquel should be an over-the-counter sleep aid. Xanax for my flight, Xanax for my meeting, Xanax to deal with my kids, my husband, my life.

Percocet for a sprained ankle, Percocet for a broken toe, Percocet because "it's the only thing that works!"

American medicine has become the justification of illness, not the treatment of it.

You wonder why your doctor can't see you today? Because of the fifty other people like you who called in the last hour with a minor viral illness. Because your doctor now has to see thirty-five patients in the same amount of time they used to see fifteen.

You wonder why they don't want to spend any time with you? *Because they can't.* There is no time. Because insurance rates have gone sky-high while insurance reimbursement is capped, and it sucks. You think your doctor is getting rich off of you? Some HMO contracts reimburse at around ten dollars per patient. Why? Because patients see the doctor ten times a year instead of two or three. Because after those ten visits, they buy fifty medications. Because at 300 pounds and seventy years old, most people would've been dead twenty years ago but now they'll be alive for another twenty.

When not tending to national emergencies, my home was the urgent care. Urgent Care, the bottom of the hair-clogged drain that is the cesspool of modern medicine. What began as a great idea, a bridge between primary care and the emergency room, has morphed into the fast food of medical care. It has completely removed the personal responsibility from people as patients, as parents, as spouses, and as children of the elderly.

Don't like being relegated to seeing the PA or Nurse Practitioner? Too bad, get used to it. The profession that used to command both salary and respect has become a losing proposition. *There won't be any primary care doctors in twenty years.*

Welcome to the death of American medicine.
Now, may I take your order?

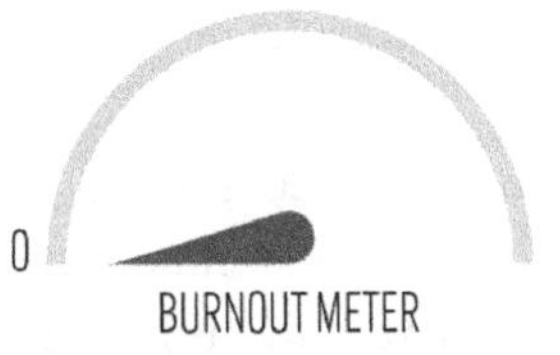

Moosecock 20/20

Wellington Emergency Department, Florida 2005

Moosecock: Pain-in-the-ass male patient.

Before I met my mentor, Mike, I noticed a young and clearly pregnant girl bickering with her mom in the waiting room. I thought she might be in the wrong place and set that thought aside as I popped through the doorway to introduce myself to whoever had the privilege of mentoring me over the next six weeks.

I nervously ducked through the main ER in a pair of too-new scrubs and a stethoscope around my neck, trying to appear as little student-like as I could. Across the hall, the "Fast Track" section of the emergency room beckoned. A dumping ground for every bleeding patient, injury, or nebulous abdominal pain that could be anything from a Urinary Tract Infection (UTI) to a surgical admission. It was not the in-and-out promise made to the public, but certainly the expectation of the then ER director. Appropriately but deceivingly named, it was indeed the fast track to insanity and burnout for any PA. The goal: turn over six beds *every hour* of a ten- to twelve-hour shift.

Standing silently with a schmucky grin, I waited as Mike finished up a few orders and laughed with the nurse.

He finally turned to acknowledge my "Hi, I'm your new student."

He met me with a thick Long Island accent and all the enthusiasm of a teen Chipotle employee being asked for extra guac. I astutely asked him if he was from New York in an effort to potentially bond, and instead he grunted and pointed for me to sit. While I did my best to hang on to every word of his instructions, I couldn't help but notice the pregnant girl being led into a room by the triage nurse, followed closely by her mom.

Mike glanced at her chart (yes, paper charts on rusty metal clipboards back then), shrugged and said, "Back pain in a sixteen-year-old, greeeeaaaat."

"She's pregnant," I chuckled. "Did you see her?"

Before he could raise his eyebrows in curiosity, we heard a life-changing scream. Scrambling to open Door 6, we found two women *in shock*. The cross-bearing mom, who apparently had been in complete denial about her daughter's pregnancy, hunched over in prayer. And our sixteen-year-old, tears pouring out of a frightened face, who had pushed her newborn into the waiting arms of a dirty toilet.

My street CV includes delivering three babies in the field, plus my own firstborn. This is four more than most medics ever will, period. It is one of the most ass-puckering calls any medic can receive. If you're picturing Dwight Schrute dropping a watermelon, you're not far off. It's a level of panic far beyond cardiac arrest. Even with the experience of having delivered a cord-dangled and barely breathing baby in a Yonkers apartment under my belt, I remember the dread of being called for a subway pregnancy on the Upper East Side. As we hit the switches and drove the bus

   American Triage

(ambulance) more recklessly than usual, my partner, Steve, reminded me to grab the rarely seen OB kit when we got there.

"Oh, we're not bringing the OB kit," I said.

Steve was a little taken aback as we routinely brought all our bags just in case the dispatcher hadn't been given accurate details. "What do you mean, why not?"

"We're not delivering a fucking baby on the subway. Then stair chairing them both up three flights of shitty steps backwards, all while hoping they're both okay," I said. "Nope, we're going to boogie down there with the chair, and unless I hear 'daddy,' this kid ain't coming out until we hit Lenox Hill."

Steve grabbed the O2 bag out of habit, and we jumped down the steps, seat-belted our relieved patient whose water had broken, and proceeded to carry her up the three flights and get her to the ER before there was any crowning. Drenched in subway and ambulance sweat, we felt like we had won some sort of sick CrossFit event.

This is why I have four, not five.

Regardless, I've always had a soft spot for pregnant patients. Not only the responsibility of suddenly being tasked with two potential emergencies, but the incumbent panic most mothers instinctively feel when a pregnancy is at risk. My favorite nurse, Becca, would even chastise me for the flood of orders and concern that accompanied pregnancy workups.

Back at the toilet, the odds of two former New York medics who had both delivered babies in the field being on shift together in a South Florida ER were pretty slim. Pretty damn fortunate for that baby as well. This was hardly an at-home doula water birth.

Gloves on, we scooped the eerily silent baby from the toilet and kept her level with mom, who was now on the stretcher. Mike conjured up an OB kit, and we suctioned and stimulated the newborn, hopeful that she hadn't aspirated any toilet water. You hear the word *stat* a bunch on medical shows. If ever there was a fucking stat call to OB, this was it.

I clamped and Mike cut the cord, hoping to control any bleeding and keep "our" baby breathing. He looked up briefly for reassurance, but I had nothing to offer but steady hands. He suctioned her mouth, then her nose again while I dried her back and still-damp hair puffs. Trying desperately to stimulate a reflexive cough or cry, I grabbed another universal white, pink, and blue blanket, rubbing her back and feet quickly and forcefully. A best-guess balance between hurting a stranger's newborn child and wishing enough discomfort to provoke life.

"I don't love her color."

"No, still a little blue."

"IS OB FUCKING READY?!!"

Mike's plea understating what was at stake for us both. His job in the balance, and me, knowing I might fail to save a baby.

In my arms.

On my first day.

Ear-piercing cries and a spasmodic clench.

One of the rare times you love to hear a newborn scream, her wails cleared a path like a siren. Mike released the stretcher brake, and I steered towards the ER elevators. We safely delivered baby and her mom to the experts upstairs, all gowned and ready to go.

And that was our introduction to each other.

Over the next twenty weeks, Mike taught me how to become a good emergency PA. I went from sewing stuffed animals to sewing lips and every other body part. How to read X-rays. How to pop dislocated fingers back into place. When he said "Let's run it by the doc," he meant let's punt this fucking case so we don't kill somebody or get sued.

And most importantly, he taught me the term *Moosecock*.

Heavy duty training, indeed.

And here we are twenty years later, both out of medicine.

The best PA I ever saw or worked with. Over that time, our wives and kids became friends. We helped each other get jobs and helped each other get through shifts with the promise of a Stoli Vanil or a Goose and cranberry. He lured me unsuspectingly to Miami to help him move a four-billion-gallon fish tank and all the water that came with it! And he was smart enough to get out of medicine before I did. At the time I questioned his decision, and later it inspired me.

Thank you, Moosecock.

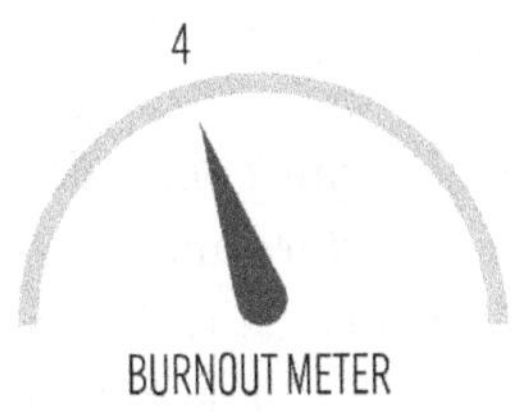

Cut Me Mick

Palm Beach Gardens, Florida 2013

I walk into the exam room to find a young and grimy look-ing kid, barely in his twenties. Unbothered by my appear-ance. Texting and snarling.

I risk the interruption.

"Hi, what brings you in today, dude?"

Looking up from his cell phone, annoyed.

"Oh, I'm not here for me. Didn't the front desk tell you?"

Returning to his phone, like he had just asked for a coffee refill.

"Tell me what?"

"Oh, I'm a Cut Man."

"A *cut man*? Can you maybe expand on that a little?"

Finally invested in the con, he lights up.

"Yeah, you know, for boxers. I have a fight this Friday actually."

"Like Mickey from *Rocky*?"

Blank stare. Ughh.

Obviously, this punk is not familiar with The Italian Stallion.

"Like I was saying, I have a fight in a few days, and I like to be prepared."

Where the hell is this going? Florida is not exactly a hotbed of pugilistic performance.

"But, YOU'RE not actually fighting, right?"

"No, I'm the Cut Man! I need to be prepared for bleeding, like, uncontrollable bleeding."

"Always good to be prepared."

"So, what I need from you, doc, is *cocaine*. Pharmaceutical-grade cocaine, preferably."

Would I be so insolent as to carry any other kind?

Wow, this guy has really done his research. While it is true that on the rarest of occasions ER docs and surgeons use cocaine to stop nosebleeds, I don't think boxing licenses their corner men to dump coke on participants' faces in the event of a gushing head wound.

"You think an urgent care has a pharmacy? And in that pharmacy, locked up behind the nitroglycerin, is cocaine?"

This isn't going as well as he had hoped.

"They told me at the front desk you could help me out."

This is probably true. Our staff is instructed to never turn *anyone* away.

"Tell you what. Wait here . . ."

I disappear into the lab where we keep, not Schedule II drugs, but the ENT kit. Returning to the exam room, I make a show of opening the tackle box.

From under the stacked yellow trays filled with silver nitrate, gauze, and Steri-Strips, I pull out a squeeze bottle.

"Here's your answer," I say, handing it to him.

"The fuck is this! Afrin?!!"

"You got it! Great vasoconstrictor. Good luck this Friday!"

"I can't use this shit!"

Believe me, I respect a high-level executive pitch for pharmaceutical grade narcotics as much as the next PA, but I have to draw the line somewhere.

"Tell you what. Why don't I call the police and you can explain the predicament the Florida Boxing Commission has put you in."

He feigns outrage as he hops off the table and turns to me with one last plea.

"So where am I going to get coke from?!!"

Good question, my friend, good question.

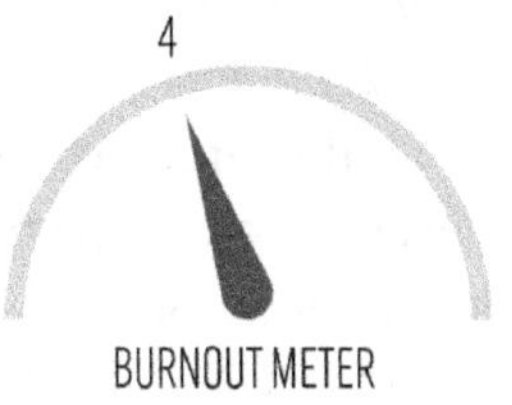

Antiscience

Palm Beach County, Florida 2000s

Pseudoscience is disturbing enough. Ideas presented as valid scientific beliefs that are not grounded in any scientific method, and are so baseless that they can be hard to disprove. Practicing medicine places you into the center ring as a punching bag for these beliefs. This type of thinking ranges from the essentially harmless (e.g., I loaded up on Vitamin C, I caught a cold from being in the rain) to the totally reckless (e.g., vaccines cause autism). Pseudoscience is so pervasive through everything from oral myths to social media that we encounter it on an all-too-frequent basis.

In his book *Antifragile*, Nassim Nicholas Taleb describes this condition as something that benefits from randomness or shocks to the status quo. As it applies to medicine (something he dedicates an entire chapter to), he writes:

> *The hidden costs of health care are largely in the denial of antifragility . . . the attempt by humans to*

Wrapped in his antifragility argument is a discussion of iatrogenics, the inadvertent adverse effects caused by medical treatment or advice. Or more simply, a process in which the cure is sometimes more harmful than the disease. Taleb correctly points out these processes which continue to fragilize our society. Shockingly, American medicine has cultivated a process by which its own patients request iatrogenesis.

No surgical patient would willingly request that their doctor leave a blood-soaked sponge lodged in their abdominal cavity long after they've been sewn up, or to have the wrong leg operated on. My own GI doctor forced a colonoscopy on me before he would band my hemorrhoids, knowing full well that given my age and family history I had no chance of having colon cancer. The risk of him rupturing the walls of my colon were far greater than the chance he would discover disease, but he ordered it anyway.

These are iatrogenic examples. Our patients however, continuously request medications that theoretically offer much more potential harm than value for them; they *demand* to be treated this way.

Therein lies much of the dilemma of practicing medicine in this country.

Think of a common example in football. Throwing a pass is said to have one potential good outcome, but a few bad ones. The pass could be completed for either a positive gain or even a touchdown. The negative outcomes could

---

[1] Nassim Nicholas Taleb, *Antifragile: Things That Gain from Disorder* (Random House, 2012).

be an incompletion, a sack, or the ultimate negative conse-
quence of a turnover via interception.

This is analogous to patients popping into my urgent
care within the first forty-eight hours of cold symptoms
and requesting antibiotics. Sure, they might actually have
a bacteria-induced illness such as strep and receive proper
treatment. More likely however, we are rolling the dice
with the following scenarios as we shift towards patient-
centered practice.

First, we hope that the antibiotic simply placates our
patients while symptomatic treatment and natural immunity bring them back to health. Second, we add to the regional resistance rates of that particular antibiotic by writing it unnecessarily. Third, we get an increasing number
of callbacks when our patients suddenly can't stop going to
the bathroom due to the proliferation of C. diff (see "Turd
Milkshake"). And last, we contribute to the creation of new
superbugs like CRE (Carbapenem-resistant Enterobacteriaceae), leaving ourselves with less and less viable antibiotic alternatives for treatment of new illnesses.

But remember, this is what our patients want, and we
have a term for this phenomenon.

Antiscience.

Antiscience is a rejection of modern science and the
scientific method. This isn't grounded skepticism that
questions whether or not medications do more harm than
good. This is a rejection of a rejection. There are many
studies that conclude antibiotics are unnecessary for common infections, but we are considered uncaring if we don't
prescribe medications against what we know to be scientific standards.

A recent study by the Infectious Diseases Society of
America revealed that up to 98% of sinus infections are

viral, but no less than 90%.[2] This means that for the twenty cases of self-diagnosed sinusitis which I'll treat tomorrow, probably one, maybe zero, but not more than two of those patients should receive antibiotics. However, patients not only pre-select their diagnosis, they commonly pre-select the antibiotic they believe will fix them. The same study urges us if we must treat sinusitis, to stick with Augmentin, not plain amoxicillin or other medications. This is due to increased resistance rates. But when I mention to patients in our particular area that the medicine they crave, a Z-Pak, has a 38% resistance rate[3] to the most common causes of sinusitis, they laugh.

"I've taken it lots of times and *my* body isn't resistant to it."

Now we're entertaining a combination of antiscience *and* pseudoscience. They have asked for treatment with a medication that in my urgent care has at best a 6.2% chance of working if we're using their diagnosis. Even if they are afflicted with a true bacterial sinusitis, they want a medication that fails almost 40% of the time!

So what's going on here? Do patients knowingly request antibiotics despite football fields of studies dispelling them of their benefits? Refer back to Taleb's comments about comfort. There is something much more insidious at play.

---

[2] Anthony W. Chow et al., "Executive Summary: IDSA Clinical Practice Guideline for Acute Bacterial Rhinosinusitis in Children and Adults," *Clinical Infectious Diseases* 54, no. 8 (April 15, 2012): 1041–45, https://doi.org/10.1093/cid/cir1043.

[3] Florida Department of Health, "Summary of Antimicrobial Resistance Surveillance," *Florida Department of Health Report*, n.d., https://www.floridahealth.gov/diseases-and-conditions/disease-reporting-and-management/disease-reporting-and-surveillance/data-and-publications/_documents/2009-section4.pdf.

Americans *like* being sick.

We have created a culture around illness, around taking our kids to the urgent care or emergency room as a post-Walmart event. Does a four-year-old even know what a headache is? Does a twenty-five-year-old really think that they're having a cardiac event when they tell me they are having chest pain?

Our patients often don't want the truth. However, we must be complicit in the charade. We must sometimes practice bad medicine in order to be available to practice good medicine. Prescriptions for antibiotics, muscle relaxers, and cough syrup provide "proof of illness." This is the desired outcome:

"Hey, Bob, how are you feeling?"

"Not too good, Jimbo."

"Did you go to the urgent care?"

"Yeah, they put me on a Z-Pak."

"A Z-Pak? Wow, you must be really sick!"

The eyes get even wider when steroids are on the table. "Wow, you think I need steroids, Doc? It's that bad, huh? Wait till I tell Jimbo I'm on the juice!"

So never mind the extensive warnings on the CDC homepage. Never mind a little science. Never mind that people somehow used to live before penicillin was discovered. Perhaps the words of my coworker will stick with us the next time we want to overtreat the common cold.

"A little dirt never hurt."[4]

---

[4] Note: Portions of this chapter originally appeared in the November 2014 issue of *JAAPA*.
Adam Axler, "Antiscience," *JAAPA* 27 (11): 1-2, https://doi.org/10.1097/01.JAA.0000455660.50166.8a.

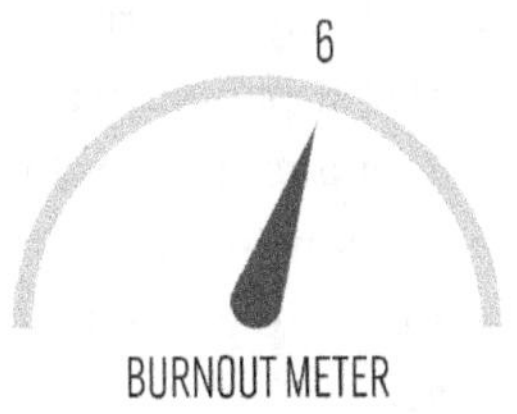

I Put Yogurt in My Vagina

South Florida 2012

I guess the title gives away the punch line, but let me backtrack a little. Weekends at the urgent care are not only busy, but bizarre. However, they are also neatly divided between mornings and afternoons. In the morning, we have a line of patients waiting at the door as if we were giving away free bags of gold or were the newest club in town. While annoying, the bulk of the legitimate patients for the day will come from this group. Ear infections or a strep throat that woke a child, the first chance to see a doctor after a busy workweek, or weekend warriors who sprained an ankle in their Old Man Leagues.

The afternoon patients? Not so much.

My general feeling is that if you can't make it to the clinic by noon, *then you ain't that sick*. You've gone out to breakfast, taken the kids to their soccer game, or hit the mall first. Stopping in to see us is an afterthought on a shopping list, not an urgent visit. The other side of that are patients who are *truly* sick. They literally can't get out of bed until three o'clock. CHFers and COPDers (congestive heart failure and chronic obstructive pulmonary disease) who can't breathe, a patient having chest pain who should've called 9-1-1, or a septic child whose parents have done everything wrong, now popping in one-by-one in the hopes that they won't have to go to the hospital.

They are all wrong.

This is about the time I implement my Z-Pak or ER triage system. If your complaint can't be readily treated with a Z-Pak or an ace wrap, then you are setting sail for the emergency room, or at least a specialist referral. No lab work, no MRI script, no fancy in-depth evaluation that you should have consulted your primary care doctor for months ago. You want answers today? Go to the hospital. Could it be this, could it be that? Sure, could be. Z-Pak. Next.

Sometimes our patients are kind enough to throw out subtle hints as to which branch of the triage tree we should lean towards. For example, we have the "Bed Head Sign." Coined by a former ER doc, a positive bed head sign is never a good thing. Usually seen in the elderly, an unkempt coif with multiple strands poking in assorted directions means that this patient was flat on their face for hours, or unable to move. If you are too sick to find a minute to comb your hair or put on your hat, then you are too sick to be here.

Along those same lines is the "Positive Pajama Sign" (also known as bathrobe sign). I'm not talking about toddlers strutting around in their Superman Underoos. No, I'm talking about fully grown adults wearing pajamas in the middle of the afternoon to a professional medical practice. The implication here is simple. Either you are so sick that you couldn't get dressed, or that somehow you think your provider will give you better care while dressed in your bunny slippers, out of sympathy. I can tell you that whichever the reason, it's not going to be fixed with a Z-Pak.

But as the afternoon progresses into evening, and the inevitable search for a "full moon" by one of the nurses commences, the truly bizarre becomes possible. As I finish telling yet another New York tourist, whose son is still garbed in a swimsuit and sunburned to a crisp, that indeed sharing water bottles with his strep-infected sister was a bad idea, I sign up for the next chart.

Chief complaint? *Vaginal Discharge.*

GYN services have actually become almost obsolete in our current setting. We don't even carry cultures to perform routine swabs, and gonorrhea and chlamydia are more accurately tested through urine now. So there is never truly a reason for me to perform a pelvic exam ever again, other than to look for and not find "your missing tampon." There is nothing a few prescriptions and a follow-up can't handle. So I was caught slightly off guard when I entered and saw what appeared to be a pleasant lady in her sixties.

And by pleasant, I mean *crazy.* When I made the mistake of probing about the nature of the discharge, instead of an answer, I was handed a paper-clipped research packet.

"So, this doesn't feel like a yeast infection?"

"A yeast infection? Well, maybe, except for the fact that my boyfriend of two years slept with a *heroin addict prostitute* without telling me."

Whoa, whoa, whoa, whoa.

"Oh, you don't think it's a yeast infection?"

"I've been doing a lot of research."

As I could see.

"I think I have trichomoniasis. I've been oozing for

about a week."

Odd that she would pick only that one, but okay, I'll play along.

"Sure, we can treat that. I'll write you a few prescriptions and have you follow up with your OB tomorrow for some formal cultures . . ."

"You're not going to do that now?"

"No, we don't even have the swabs to test you. But I'm sure that your OB can help you out."

"I have to see another doctor?"

"Yes, I'm not a gynecologist."

"Oh, well what about the yeast?"

"I thought you said it was trich?"

"I think it might be both. But I've been using yogurt."

"Good, yogurt is good."

"But I don't think that I've been using a big enough tube."

Oh no.

"Because I'm having a hard time getting enough in."

Yep.

"Should I be using a bigger . . ."

"OK, that's enough. So, you're telling me that you're not eating the yogurt but . . ."

"Eating it? No, I'm putting it in my vagina!"

"And who told you to do that?"

"Oh, my friend or somebody."

"Your gynecologist perhaps?"

"No, I don't think so."

"No, *I* don't think so either. Why don't you stop doing that, it may be making things worse. Try *eating* it next time."

"So, I still need to see a gynecologist?"

Yes, bring your research packet. Don't forget to mention

*the prostitute. And whatever you do, don't hit the grocery
store on the way to the appointment.*

As I walk to my car in the pitch black, there is no illumina-
tion from a full moon, only the strange darkness of weekend medicine.

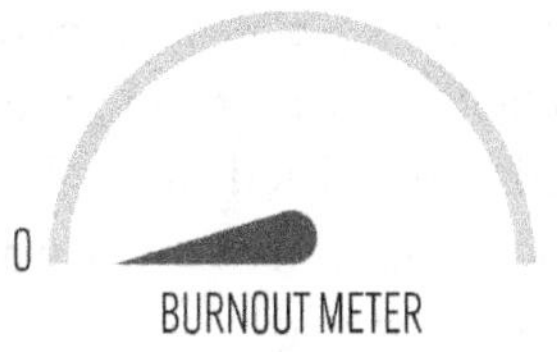

The Hanging Strangers

Manhattan, NY 2000

He pushed down his nausea and made his way back to the sidewalk. He was shaking all over, with revulsion—and fear. Why? Who was the man? Why was he hanging there? What did it mean? And—why didn't anybody notice?[5]

—Philip K. Dick, "The Hanging Stranger"

I noticed.

We kill the sirens and jump the dark. Two cruisers beat us to the apartment, so we slide past a half-open door into a poorly renovated multiunit. Stale weed and still-burning cigarettes hover as we rush to our patient's bedroom.

Shock doesn't affect everyone in the same way. A roommate paces the hallway and mumbles, mumbles.

Why won't he get up, why won't he get up.

He won't move. He won't answer me.

Why won't he get up . . .

---

[5] Philip K. Dick, "The Hanging Stranger," in *Science Fiction Adventures*, ed. Harry Harrison (Future Publications, 1953), 122-136.

The police officers shuffle to the side and I can now see the slumped body. Ghostly ash with mottled purple hickeys and cheeks. The body has been in the closet for hours. Maybe days? Piled and twisted into a little corner like a human marionette. Unnatural in every way.

But there's only one string.

Cheap corded rope, tied tightly but with a slippable, amateurish knot around the boy's neck. The other end wraps over a lacquered closet rod between worn sweaters and a wrinkled dress shirt. While the officers alert the coroner, my partner calmly radioes in the "10-83," the code for *patient pronounced dead*, to dispatch. I drop my EMS bag and make a temporary seat.

I alternate between taking in mental screenshots of the death scene and holding my head with eyes squeezed shut. I have seen suicides before. Mangled jumpers smashed on Upper East Side streets. Barely recognizable last-second subway dives. Heroin ODs laid out between toilet and tub, tubing and needle still intact.

But as I look at this poor kid, who might be my age or just a year or two younger, I'm struck with a terrifying sadness. Transmuting from whatever unlivable world he needed to leave to an afterthought on my run report.

What hurts me?

What haunts me?

He really wanted to die.

This is no belt asphyxiation kink gone wrong. No, at any time he could have simply stood up or pulled the knot loose. A hard tug would have either snapped the rope or the rod it was tied to. A forceful kick would have knocked the closet's false wood backing right into the next room. This is an executed plan.

Fighting every last second to *not* breathe.

Suffering on top of death.

Fuck me.

You see it? You see it hanging there? A man's body! A dead man![6]
—Philip K. Dick

I did see him.

Working my Lenox Hill double on the 10 Young bus, the call comes over from dispatch as an unconscious (UNCON) patient. A nebulous catchall for everything from sleeping drunks to diabetic comas. We hit the lights and head south towards the river, covering for a displaced Cornell EMS unit.

On the Upper East Side, between 68th and 73rd, there are a few pre-war buildings where architects did their best to screw with future paramedics. While the ever-wet brick or stone entrance steps are always an obstacle, opening the front door can reveal anything from a rent-controlled palace to *Jumanji*. Some steps wide enough for four medics to stair chair a patient down six flights, and others so tight we have to lift patients over railings at awkward angles with two bags strapped to our shoulders.

Dented doors with loose or missing apartment numbers belie what's behind them. Sometimes cockroaches sharing water bowls with cats in a patient's oblivious squalor. Other doors open to dated but splendorous speakeasies. Art and books and crystal highball glasses everywhere. So anything is possible as we carry our heavy packs to the UNCON on the top floor.

------

[6] Philip K. Dick, "The Hanging Stranger."

The single room is cavernous by NYC standards, with high arching ceilings and latticed beams. Except for a kicked-over wooden chair, the floor is barren. The hanging stranger splits the sky in an open robe and soiled underwear. The smell piercing and morbid.

The old man had made a real noose and knew that when he stepped off the chair there was no going back. Dependent lividity, pooling blood. A simpler plan, one that only years later can I forgive myself for thinking, *Hey, this hanging was better than that one.*

Shock doesn't affect everyone in the same way.

"10 Young" . . . *beep.*

"Go, 10 Young."

"10-83."

"Copy. 10-83."

Dr. T

Boynton Beach, Florida 2009

Twenty-eight to three.

What I had envisioned as a lengthy career in the ER came to a stunning halt, working an overnight with the newest attending. Aside from handing out free Diet Cokes from the doctors' lounge to my coworkers, I hated everything about those twelve-hour shifts. And on this particular night, they stuck me with a doctor who had never managed the ER by herself. A newbie PA with less than a year of experience to help us get to morning.

As charts kept piling up on my desk, I wondered what the fuck was going on. I checked the tracker and noticed that I was assigned to *every* patient in the ER. I had overheard the mid-shift, double-boarded doctor say he would be available by phone all night if needed, before he abandoned us, but his comment wasn't directed towards me. I later learned that the nurses were instructed to not bring any case other than a heart attack or stroke to the overnight doc, who sat nervously at her station as I drowned in orders and procedures.

By the time the sun and my relief finally came, the score was 28–3. I had seen twenty-eight patients, including two admissions, while the ER doc had sat on a total of three patients over twelve hours.

Again: 28–3.

Drinking in large gulps of an iced Dunkin' to stay awake for the long drive home, I realized that nobody gave a shit about what happened overnight. And the hospital was perfectly willing to let me ruin my career on any given day. As I showered off the ER stench and dove into bed for the first time in over twenty-four hours, I thought, *no fucking way.* No fucking way was I going to let my first job be my last, handed a shit sandwich to choke down a lawsuit or a tarnished resume.

Especially for this place, complete with affairs, dope stealing, beyond-the-norm antisemitism, and an ER manager who told me to go fuck myself after I asked him what a ninety-eight-year-old with a brain bleed was doing in my Fast Track.

So I left that ER with much less than the ninety-day notice required, but since there are no laws in Florida, I knew any threats would be as idle as the attending who dangled me over career suicide. The first urgent care (started concurrently with my ER gig) was complicit in Florida's reputation as a pill mill, with the owner actively "recommending" prescriptions in real time. I didn't play ball and quickly left before one of my patients OD'd. The second urgent care was an escape hatch from the ER, the easiest job I've ever had, aside from the owners lying about providing me with liability coverage (kind of important in one of the most litigious states in the country). And the third was run by a doctor more interested in playing poker at the dog track or online than taking care of patients.

But don't say I'm not an optimist.

I walked past the Christmas decorations and marbled front desk into my fourth urgent care job in three years since graduating from PA school. It was the first time I met Sheryl, Dr. Thompson. The doctor my own wife, Lori, would eventually refer to as my "work wife." Before there was an urgent care on every corner and inside every CVS or Walmart, UC life was *busy.* I saw *46* patients on our first shift together and the clinic saw over 100 patients that day.

It was clear, as I endured a light grilling throughout the day that any PA fairly endures from the doctors who have to co-sign their charts (making sure that you are not killing patients behind closed doors and then signing their careers away), that Sheryl had an innate kindness and brilliance that permeated the entire clinic. The combative pride of "don't tell me how to do the same job you're doing" between PA and doctor was easily allayed, and I left that first thirteen-hour day exhausted, but feeling utterly appreciated and welcomed.

Finally, a chance for the personal and professional fulfillment that had pushed me to jump from medic to physician assistant.

Over almost fifteen years and hundreds of shifts with Dr. T across clinics in three cities, I learned more about good medicine and human empathy than all of my other days on shift combined. When my daughter had her first true respiratory illness complete with retractions and wheezing, I sought out Sheryl, not our pediatrician. She calmly placed a purple dinosaur mask over Sammi's face for a nebulizer treatment, and reassured her as she drank an oral steroid that made most kids puke. I was never offended when patients asked if they "could see Dr. T instead," because that's a choice I would make for my own family. Hardly a shift went by where a patient being escorted out couldn't be overheard saying to her, "Can't you be my regular doctor?"

As my motivation devolved from competing with Sheryl for the highest patient satisfaction scores in the company to barely being able to force myself to return to shift after lunch, she remained resolute in her belief that taking care of people in any environment was still noble, or at least, valuable. Perhaps Max Von Sydow summed it up best as he explained to Robert Redford why he had not killed him in *Three Days of the Condor*:

"There is no cause. There's only yourself. The belief is in your own precision."[7]

I don't want to minimize the difficulty of maintaining the highest levels of professionalism and acumen throughout decades in patient care. As if to say anyone who "really got into medicine for the right reasons" can deal with anything.

No, that's bullshit.

The burnout rate in emergency medicine isn't high, it's *100%*.

The hordes of boomers who plague Florida's urgent cares for six-month stretches are not shy about racist or misogynistic overtones, and Sheryl has endured them both. So while you should be worried and wary that our healthcare system could force someone like me out, someone who also got into medicine for all the right reasons and took on six figures of debt to do so while deciding a six-figure salary wasn't worth the daily pain, you should also be thankful.

Thankful that on a random South Florida day, your

---

[7] *Three Days of the Condor*, directed by Sydney Pollack (Paramount Pictures, 1975), VHS.

aging mother or injured child might have the privilege of stumbling into the right urgent care and being cared for by Dr. T. And instead of complaining about your fifty-dollar copay or twenty-minute wait time, why don't you fucking say "thank you" to someone who should have given up on you and medicine years ago.

The Timeline: Part 1

0800:

Arrive at work. Lenox Hill Hospital located at E. 77th between Lexington and Park in Manhattan.

Strutting to work, past the gross Gristedes, past H&H Bagels, the sun bounces off of my twenty-seven-year-old biceps in my Lenox Hill polo as I make the six-block journey from my Upper East Side walkup. Shining off my cool Arnette sunglasses, as much the currency of NYC medics as Patrick Bateman's bone-colored business card. I stand out among even the most tailored-suited clones with my EMS bag swinging over my shoulder, garnering head nods and a respect that makes leaving my hometown fire department a lot more palatable.

No "narc pouch" needed to run 10 Frank, a Basic Life Support (BLS) unit in the NYC 9-1-1 system. This still means working shootings, stabbings, and high-speed car crashes; hardly a day off. The even-numbered units are stationed on the East Side, odd numbers on the West Side. The higher the number, the farther uptown your area. Lenox Hill has the 10 and 11 units. It's the busiest of all my shifts, a sixteen-hour double. I greet my partner Steve, always edgy but prepared, with a friendly smile. He mentions during our morning checks that our EMS radios are only putting out static.

It's September 11th, eight o'clock. 2001.

0848–0849:

Radios tuned to Manhattan Central frequency.

FDNY EMS Unit:

"Zero One Charlie for the priority."

"Go ahead, Zero One Charlie."

"A plane just crashed into the World Trade Center."

"10-5?"

"Yeah, right!!!" (laughter)

Annoying Nextels chirp from our hips every few seconds, too often.

Steve comments that planes have hit the WTC before, but we both feel something's terribly wrong.

Of all the days for our portables to not work. Even though Lenox Hill is a private hospital, any unit working in the NYC 9-1-1 system is under the supervision of FDNY EMS (New York City Fire Department Bureau of Emergency Medical Services). They are their own department, completely independent of the firefighters. So any communication issues or mechanical problems that might take you out of service have to be cleared with an FDNY captain or "boss."

We head over to the closest FDNY operations center, Metropolitan Hospital, previously best known for George Costanza's sponge bath incident. We need an FDNY captain to physically exchange our radios so they don't think we're napping in Central Park or roaming forty blocks out of our area.

Steve and I are already antsy, waiting for dispatch to belt out a thick cadence of regular jobs into the ether before they materialize on our radios or bus screens as our assignments. Metro is twenty blocks north of our area; we'd be scrambling back to post up across from the Guggenheim before being plucked for yet another Randall's Island psych call. Foolishly thinking *that* might be the clusterfuck of the day.

Then:

"A plane just crashed into the World Trade Center!!"

Without hesitation, the captain cranks up the squelch.

"Confirmed."

0903:

At Metropolitan Hospital. Still waiting for FDNY "boss" to exchange radios. Hear our coworker Tom say, *"10 Oscar, 10 Oscar, another . . ."*

Numb to the waves of cardiac arrests, shootings, fatal accidents, and subway suicides that chirp across EMS radio daily, this hits *very* different. Having recently come from a suburban Cleveland fire department, I had only worked two or three cardiac arrests. Those deaths sat with us an entire week, firefighters losing members of their hometown. At Lenox Hill, some of the medics come from units where they work two or three arrests *per shift*, distractions between feedings at Ranch One or Ray's Original. Once, I even told Steve to stop eating his pizza in front of a dead suicide jumper.

But this isn't the nice, slow buzz of who's going to tube (intubate) and who's going to run the Lifepak 12 in case we need to shock. This is straight pre-5-hour-Energy bodega ephedrine with a Red Bull chaser (a common medic cocktail). A fear of the unknown, not felt since the Oklahoma City bombing, jacks us with a rush.

Playing firefighter in a low-volume suburban department is one thing. Being transported to the alien planet of NYC to run EMS calls all day is another. I thought I was on a one-year free agent contract with the Yankees, on loan from Cleveland. One year (*which turned into five*) to let Lori live her New York dream, and for me to live a surreal existence as a medic in NYC. To pay two grand a month for a fourth-floor walkup because it has exposed brick! To drive an ambulance down the sidewalk in Times Square to work a double shooting. To work ODs in the Plaza Hotel and the subway at W. 79th and Broadway.

So, I thought I was long past innocent, when I hear Tom's voice.

At twenty-seven years old, hear the end of my childhood.

"*. . . plane has hit the second tower.*"

0906–0924

Steve annihilates 2nd Ave., hits 79th and cuts through Central Park over to the West Side. We look for any excuse to get assigned to the Mass Casualty Incident (MCI). Under normal circumstances dispatch assigns jobs, but New York is under attack and they are lost. Redirect at W. 52nd. Decide to linger, wait for our next chance. Cell phones dead.

Unmarked Crown Vics race past us to disaster while dispatch makes shit up, randomly assigning units to join or not join them.

What the fuck are we doing?

Literally.

Should we find Steve's dad working in the towers and get him to safety? Is that even possible? Do I know anyone in the towers, Jesus! Did we just lose our jobs? Do we care? *Phones are dead.* Lori is in the air.

Am I going to risk my life for strangers in a city I had to be dragged to?

No/Maybe/No.

Take a deep breath.

Yes.

Three minutes ago, Lenox Hill Hospital employed us. Now, we are only employed in *the fight* as CITIZENS OF NEW YORK.

0950–0953:

Tower 2 collapses.

Calls come in for additional units.

Dispatch finally assigns us to the towers.

We scream lights and sirens down the West Side Highway and lie about being fifty blocks south. Eight miles from Lenox Hill, hurling past time, death, and the lives of millions of New Yorkers on our way. The Unknown straight ahead. At 90 mph, I find courage in what is left unsaid between Steve and me.

Stay together, stay alive.

1000–1008:

In place of Tower 1's top floors, a dark hole, oddly and grotesquely shaped, carved out by a passenger jetliner. Nothing could be more real or terrifying. The New York skyline forever altered. Smoke gathers, before shooting out in bursts from the side of the tower's new mouth. Insidious superheated jet fuel gets to work melting the girders, first in drips, then in vertically layered waves.

Steve and I naively press forward, so desperate to help that the cognitive dissonance of walking through the remains of the South Tower has nothing to do with the one that is currently burning down in exactly the same way.

Things keep falling from the sky.

Steve warns me to watch for debris. I pause and squint,

but can't process what I'm seeing. I squint again to spin the roulette wheel, hoping as the ball falls this time my eyes can properly focus through the sun and white smoke.

That's not debris.

It's people.

Of all the horrors I live with, this one remains the most hideous. The tower becomes a multilayer incinerator, leaving its casualties with the choice of burning alive or falling over 100 stories to their deaths. But for now, I have to set it aside. It's only ten o'clock.

"MAYDAY, MAYDAY."

The call of last resort.

I have never heard that call, a 10-fucking-13.

Have medics just died?

Ten blocks now from the first tower. Green-lit triage coded survivors run by, but for us, each step forward is like a slog through a foot of sticky Cleveland snow. The unthinkable keeps piling up.

1012–1018:

An FDNY boss directs us towards the tower. Dust-covered heads and business suits flow around us. We don our bright yellow, never-worn-before EMS helmets.

Waves of anguished faces wash past us as we wade forward looking for injured patients. More waves with bleeding forearms and thighs. Ambulatory. None stop.

Only a few blocks from the North Tower now . . .

But where are the wounded?

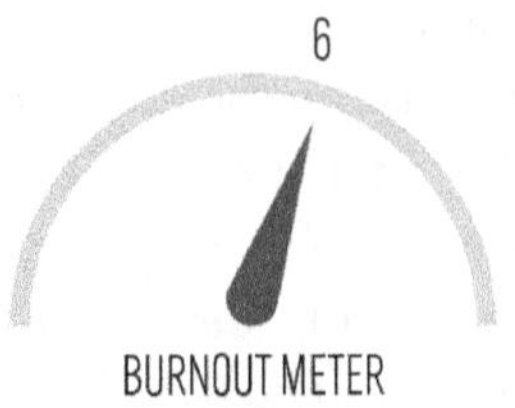

Case Study: The Ottawa Ankle Rules

Ottawa, Ontario

Probably never heard of them. Most people haven't. And when I attempt to explain them to the parents of a thirteen-year-old soccer or lacrosse player, they look at me like I'm the devil.

The rules, established by ER doctors at the Ottawa Civic Hospital in the early '90s, basically say that if you're walking after you twist your ankle, or by the time you get to the hospital, you didn't break anything. There are also the Ottawa Foot Rules, similar concept. The sensitivity of this test is almost 100%, successfully repeated over large studies.[8]

---

[8] Michelle Jenkin, Michael R. Sitler, and John D. Kelly, "Clinical Usefulness of the Ottawa Ankle Rules for Detecting Fractures of the Ankle and Midfoot," *Journal of Athletic Training* 45, no. 5 (September 1, 2010): 480–82, https://doi.org/10.4085/1062-6050-45.5.480;
Yolanda E. Gomes et al., "Diagnostic Accuracy of the Ottawa Ankle Rule to Exclude Fractures in Acute Ankle Injuries in Adults: A Systematic Review and Meta-analysis," *BMC Musculoskeletal Disorders* 23, no. 1 (September 23, 2022), https://doi.org/10.1186/s12891-022-05831-7.

The purpose of these rules is to reduce the number of mindless X-rays we take in the urgent care and ER every day, every year, for mild sprains and strains that simply need an ace wrap and an icepack (or neither).

But there are several factors at play that render these rules almost useless, outlined below:

1. The overcautious/crazy sports mom/dad who can't believe that their child has been injured playing sports.

2. The mystical "hairline" fracture.

3. The threat of litigation.

4. *Your kid is a wuss.*

Rushing your child in for X-rays after rolling an ankle playing basketball, making a slide tackle in soccer, or getting tackled in football means that *you* are probably not cut out to let your kid play sports. Sprained ankles hurt. Getting hit with a baseball in your shin hurts. If your child plays sports, they're eventually going to get hurt. Live with that truth. If you can't, don't be *Sports Dad.*

There is no such thing as a hairline fracture. If a fracture is that small, it's probably not going to show up on X-ray and unless you're the starting catcher for the LA Dodgers, it doesn't matter.

"No, it's not fractured."

"But is it broken?"

"No, that's the same thing."

"Are you sure?"

"Yes, I'm sure."

I used to work with a doc who called everything a "hairline" fracture, real popular with the staff. Splints and crutches for everyone. You know why? *Because he couldn't read X-rays.*

I know little Bobby has a sprain. You know little Bobby has a sprain. I'm pulling on his ankle, twisting it, making him walk on it. Nothing hurts. Then you turn to me and say,

"Do you really think he needs an X-ray?"

Do I think he needs one? Of course not, but you signed up for an X-ray the moment you walked in that door. Because even if there's no way in hell that Bobby has a fracture, I need to document that while you are in my presence. How do I know that your kid isn't going to slip on a step, or get hurt tomorrow doing the same thing? You rush to your lawyer and say, "That guy didn't even do an X-ray and Bobby's ankle was broken all along!" I often say to the radiology tech, "Negative X-ray going up, Room 4." That's what you're here for anyway isn't it, to irradiate your poor kid's body unnecessarily?

Finally, as a former athlete of sorts myself, and having grown up as the middle of three boys, I'll say this. For three short Jewish suburban kids, at least we weren't wusses. My older brother played Division I baseball (a venture I failed at), and my younger brother played Division I football (for Nick Saban no less).

I played through an entire season with a broken finger on my throwing hand, and my brothers played through assorted injuries that were part of growing up on frozen fields in the Midwest. We threw ice on our elbows and knees after games, and my parents never flinched at bloody body parts, golf-ball-sized contusions, and assorted limps. So when a dad brings his son in for hand pain after playing catcher, or a mom brings in her kid for sore ribs after playing flag football, what am I supposed to say?

"Yes, this could be serious, better get an X-ray."

What I have said with a straight face on several occasions is, "Perhaps your child isn't meant to play contact sports." That translates pretty directly to "your kid is a weenie, and you're only making it worse."

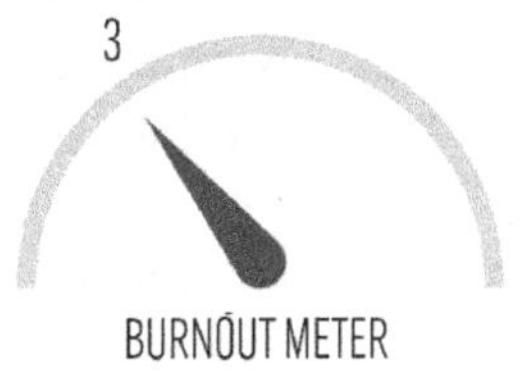

Poor Ol' Pie Face

Boynton Beach, Florida 2010

Had I not seen it before, I wouldn't have believed my eyes. An elderly woman, barely ambulatory, slowly shuffled by me into the procedure room on the arm of her friend. I quickly glanced around to see if anybody else was taking this in . . .

Her face wasn't a little bruised or a little swollen. She looked as if someone had turned her skin *inside out* and she was ready to be made into pie filling. The doc clearly didn't see her, but the PA I was working with looked at me with an expression of both shock and horror, so it was confirmed.

Yes, this woman was a human blueberry.

This is when I lovingly coined the term *Pie Face*.

Knowing full well that the odds of me sending this patient to the ER were 1000%, I clicked on her chart to ensure that I would be the one taking care of her. I had to get the scoop for myself. As I suspected, she was taking Coumadin, which is a blood thinner given to people who have had heart attacks, strokes, or who have an irregular heartbeat called atrial fibrillation (to prevent blood clots).

But Coumadin doesn't just thin the blood that goes to your brain and your heart, it thins *all* of your blood. So any time you scrape your shin, cut yourself shaving, or fall and hit something, you either bleed like crazy or look like Manny Pacquiao just beat you up for the last twelve rounds. It also greatly increases your odds of dying when you fall and hit your head because of the potential for your brain to bleed.

Oh, sure, there's been other Coumadin falls since then, but nothing like this. Half pies, quarter pies, rhubarb pies, but not a 100% blueberry pie with two stark white eyeballs staring back at me. Someone who could ask me with a straight face whether this was something that needed further evaluation.

But the mysteries of the urgent care don't end with Pie Face. No, on an almost routine basis, we are exposed to even more absurd presentations.

Take for example, *Horn Head.*

An elderly man with a squamous cell carcinoma that had grown for so long without treatment that it was actually protruding from his head in the shape of a billygoat-like horn. I resisted the urge to shout, "El Diablo!" and claimed his chart as well.

It's hard to know what the craziest part of his thinking was. That a horn growing out of the side of his head was in any way, shape, or form somehow *not cancer,* or that he could drop by the urgent care and there would be someone qualified or willing to remove it without killing him. I offer to put an axe into his skull to cut it off, but inform him that there might be some side effects . . .

I try to keep it all together, holding in both amazement

and pure disbelief while I interview this woman who looks like she's been rejected by Willy Wonka. There is nothing but deep purple across her entire face except for two white dots occasionally flashing between blinks. She proceeds to tell me how she fell yesterday, tripping in the parking lot over those damn space dividers (I suspect these things were invented by hospitals or EMS systems to cause injuries to the elderly) before face planting in the parking lot.

I calmly and casually let her finish her story and explain to me why it is that she didn't think she needed to go to the hospital when 100% of her head is a giant bruise. I wait for it because I know that it's coming, from both her and her friend. When I ask them what it is they think that I can do for them, her friend confidently says,

"We just want to make sure her head is okay."

No, your fucking head is not okay.

Just because you're not bleeding on the outside doesn't mean you're not bleeding on the inside. You look like an extra from a Wes Craven movie. I fear that every second I spend talking to you is another second that your brain is pooling with blood. I go on to explain the risks of death, of brain hemorrhage while taking a fall on Coumadin, and because no human could resist, I have to ask,

"Have you looked at yourself in the mirror? I mean, did you think that you looked okay?"

And then I wait again for the inevitable.

"So you really think I have to go to the hospital?"

I retreat to my desk to print out the transfer papers to the emergency room and give my coworkers a heads up that maybe they should look at something they may never see again. Jaw-dropping, stunned silence, and incoherent mumbles from seasoned ER docs and medics ensued.

Poor ol' Pie Face.

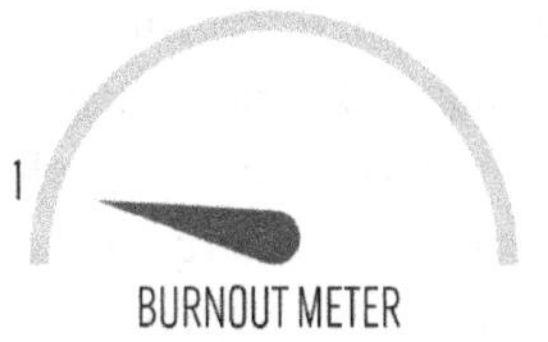

Turd Milkshake

Lenox Hill Hospital, New York City 2004

Yes, *fecal transplants*. I know, sounds like something your older brother used to threaten you with while you were sleeping. Replacing your poop with someone else's. No, it's real and it works. The process has actually been around for over fifty years (or hundreds if you count "yellow soup").[9] Whether it's placed up or down, the patient receives a "transplant" of feces from someone else, typically a family member. This is done to combat persistent diarrhea caused by overgrowth of the bacterium *Clostridioides difficile*, or C. diff. This procedure is proving to be far more effective than bombarding the GI tract with super antibiotics via IV, which works about 40% of the time.

There are several reasons why only recently a study of any sample size has been performed, despite documented

---

[9] Huan Du et al., "Fecal Medicines Used in Traditional Medical System of China: A Systematic Review of Their Names, Original Species, Traditional Uses, and Modern Investigations," *Chinese Medicine* 14, no. 31 (September 13, 2019), https://doi.org/10.1186/s13020-019-0253-x.

success over several decades. First, it's hard to find a donor. All poop isn't the same. In order for the transplant to work without passing along collateral damage in the form of disease, the fecal matter has to be screened carefully. It has to be healthy poop. Second, the actual procedure isn't exactly like getting a Botox injection. You are either "fed" a turd milkshake passed into your colon via a nasogastric tube, or the contents are passed through your rectum in the form of a fecal enema.

Delicious.

As I mentioned, not only are fecal transplants working, but they're frequently working within one or two days. The new poop restores your colonic bacteria to its previous state before the diarrhea began, and your GI system starts functioning normally again. Now, the reason I mention this is not to disgust you or to throw you off by mentioning an obscure procedure. No, I've already mentioned the real reason: C. diff.

C. diff (Clostridioides difficile), MRSA (Methicillin-Resistant Staphylococcus Aureus), and NDM-1 CRE (New Delhi metallo-beta-lactamase-1 Carbapenem-Resistant Enterobacteriaceae) are a few of our new superbugs. C. diff and MRSA used to be found only in hospital settings or in permanent nursing home residents. These infections afflicted only the chronically ill or immunosuppressed. But due to gross antibiotic abuse, these infections are now community acquired.

Illness from C. diff is caused by the destruction of our normal gut flora through antibiotic use, allowing these bacteria to overcolonize. The subsequent release of toxins causes pleasant-sounding things like pseudomembranous colitis and toxic megacolon (along with never-ending watery diarrhea). This used to be reserved for elderly, immunosuppressed patients receiving daily IV antibiotic treatments. Now you can get C. diff after your dentist puts you on clindamycin for a week.

Patients begging for unnecessary antibiotics for their viral illness often regret their choice when they call me back two days later with painful abdominal cramping and diarrhea. And then where do you go? They've already asked me for one unnecessary drug and are experiencing the unpleasant side effects of that decision. Inevitably, many patients will then ask me to change them to a second unnecessary drug that will only increase their chances of developing C. diff. When I tell them that they should stop antibiotic use altogether and wait a few more days while resting and drinking fluids, you know what comes next.

"I want my money back!"

Okay then, good luck in the hospital while you await your fecal transplant . . .[10]

MRSA, on the other hand, is everywhere. You may have read about your favorite team's quarterback needing a second surgery to "clean out an infection." That's MRSA. You may have even read about your team's entire workout facility being shut down and fumigated for a week while several players were mysteriously listed as ill on the injury report. That's also MRSA. The *MR* is the scary part. Methicillin-Resistant means resistant to penicillin and its derivatives. Penicillin used to kill everything. Now MRSA eats it for breakfast.

"Staph" (short for staphylococcus) infections have been around forever because staph is one of the normal bacteria that live on your skin. MRSA, however, is a form of

---

[10] There are now commercial fecal microbiota products such as Rebyota (administered rectally) which contain feces from healthy donors. Treatments are expensive.

super staph that was born in hospitals and nursing homes where patients were treated with strong antibiotics (some of which have since been black-boxed). Years ago, this was found only in hospitals. Now I find myself in the procedure room several times a month draining MRSA abscesses.

Not only is MRSA now community acquired, but it's virulent and extremely contagious. It's not only little old ladies who scraped their shins coming in a week later with this infection. It's young, healthy men sharing a locker room at the local gym. It's high school wrestlers who share a dirty mat. It's mechanics sharing tools at work with open, dirty wounds. And it's entire families coming in with pustules all over their bodies from sharing a bathroom and not taking proper wound precautions.

Many patients think they've been bitten by a spider or have a little rash. Three days later they have a huge cyst on their forearm or thigh. So please don't be offended when you tell me, "Hey, doc, I got this red thing on my butt" and I don't shake your hand.

When CRE was first discovered, it was killing elderly patients who contracted it at about a rate of 50%. When the CDC and even Wikipedia can only produce a few short paragraphs about something, that basically tells you that we have no idea what this thing is. The *C* stands for carbapenems, which are a group of our strongest antibiotics, the so-called "drugs of last resort." Imagine sitting in your hospital bed and your doctor telling you, "We know what's causing you to be septic, but we don't have any medicine that kills it."

This bacterium contains a new enzyme (NDM-1) that hydrolyzes carbapenems, which renders them useless. Without getting too scientific, what makes this "bug" incredibly scary is that it transfers easily between different

 American Triage

bacteria. So not only can we not kill it, but it's spreading between bacterial sources. What seemed to be initially confined to India and Pakistan has now spread throughout the world, and the number of cases is growing.[11]

What's also interesting about CRE is that one of the few drugs that *sometimes* works against it is polymyxin. The same polymyxin that you buy in over-the-counter triple-antibiotic cream and that is used in eye ointment for babies; a drug that has been around for decades.[12] There is a similar scenario with the treatment of MRSA. Long after the penicillins and quinolones stopped killing it, Bactrim, clindamycin, and doxycycline (yes, the same doxycycline your dermatologist may have treated your acne with when you were fifteen), continue to be our best weapons against MRSA. These drugs have also been around for years.

Hmmm. So we have new generations of resistant bacteria that, aside from penicillin, are only killed by the oldest antibiotics we have. Our past shining stars, Z-Pak, Levaquin, and whatever the hell is in a carbapenem aren't working, but the medication that your mother took for her UTI forty years ago is. Can we conclude from this, along with the proliferation of C. diff, that perhaps we're abusing antibiotics?

Let's go back to that hospital bed for a second. As your doctor tells you that there is no cure for the bacteria killing

---

[11] Karthikeyan K Kumarasamy et al., "Emergence of a New Antibiotic Resistance Mechanism in India, Pakistan, and the UK: A Molecular, Biological, and Epidemiological Study," *The Lancet Infectious Diseases* 10, no. 9 (August 11, 2010): 597–602, https://doi.org/10.1016/s1473-3099(10)70143-2.

[12] G. L. Xia and R. L. Jiang, "Efficacy and Safety of Polymyxin B in Carbapenem-resistant Gram-negative Organisms Infections," *BMC Infectious Diseases* 21, no. 1034 (October 4, 2021), https://doi.org/10.1186/s12879-021-06719-y.

you where you lie, you may wonder if there is hope in the near future. And the answer to that is *no*. There are almost no "new" antibiotics. What would it take to get people to stop requesting antibiotics for their common colds and mild illness? What would scare Americans, or the world for that matter, from routinely contributing to the creation of these superbugs through incessant antibiotic abuse?

I'm sure that anyone who ever had to drink another man's feces in order to feel *better*, or who had a scalpel slice into their buttocks, might feel differently than most people, but what would it take for the rest of the world? Maybe it's already here. Maybe CRE jumps from hospital beds to hotels and schools, and instead of killing 50% of the sickest patients in ICU, it kills 50% of everything. Then, and maybe then, patients might think twice before asking for a prophylactic Disney World Z-Pak "just in case."

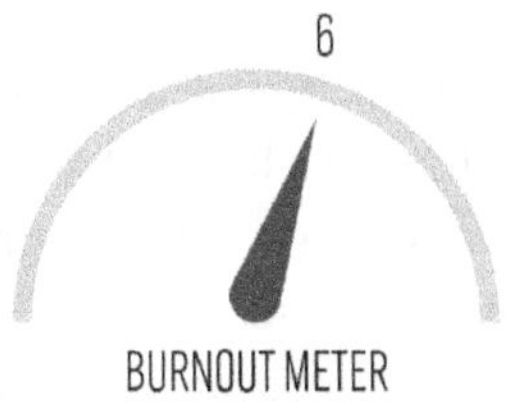

Case Study: I Forgot to Tell You Something

South Florida, 2015

You would think routine medical information like a penicillin allergy or a history of stroke would be forthcoming from my patients. You know, stuff that could potentially alter my treatment plan or potentially kill them if I'm unaware. But patients often view their medical histories as optional guidelines or even an intrusion created by the medical community to probe into their personal lives. They leak out information on an "as needed" basis determined by them, not the qualified medical professional assessing their health.

We have attempted to counteract this patient plot by creating the "Meat and Potatoes," or M&P triage process. If you are unwilling to be upfront about your entire history, then don't bore us with the color of your snot, your one episode of loose stool, or how it all started at Aunt Edna's surprise party. Strictly meat and potatoes. What brings you in today? Cough? Great, someone will be in to see you shortly.

But the chess match isn't always easy. As patients have become more accustomed to the hurry-up routine, they have craftily learned to save a bolus of complaints for their doctor or PA. Cramming in a year's worth of specialist consults into a five-minute visit.

Staring back at me with vacant eyes, between the horrendous waft of cigarette smoke and weed, was a young man I had taken care of in the past. The nurse had listed his chief complaint as "rash," but one look at his freshly inked "sleeve" tattoo and I knew that I could not escape what was about to happen.

"What can I do for you, man?"

"Well, I got this new tattoo and I think it might be infected."

"Might be?"

"OK, it's infected."

"Yep, it sure is. I'm going to get you an antibiotic and ..."

"Uh, doc, there's something else."

Fuck.

"I've been having problems with my girlfriend."

Here it comes.

"I can't always, ya know ..."

"No, I don't know. You can't always what?"

"I can't always get it hard."

"Hmmm, how long has that been going on for?"

"I don't know, a few years I think."

"Dude, you're like twenty. You've had problems getting an erection for a few years and you only mention it now because of your tattoo?"

"Maybe more like a few months."

"Any new medications you're taking, or like, maybe smoking a lot of pot?"

"Uhhh. Uhhhh. Uhhh, no?"

"Sure, okay, hmmm. This is bad. We have to get you to the urologist so you can have tests done."

"Urologist?"

"Yeah, the penis doctor."

"Oh, no, I don't need anything like that. I just need some pills."

"Ohhhh, nooooo my man. We don't get into that quick-fix type stuff when it comes to your manhood. We have to figure out what's going on with you first. Better for you *and* your girlfriend."

"Uhhh, okay."

"So head on up to the front and your prescription will be waiting for you. Don't forget to call the urologist as soon as you leave."

Yes! Another life saved. Five minutes later . . .

"He's back."

"Who's back?"

"That guy."

"Which guy?!!"

"That kid, with the thing. He said you didn't give him anything for his cold."

"What cold, he didn't mention a fucking cold!"

"He wants to talk to you."

Super pissed, I stormed out to the waiting room and told this guy to follow me back to an exam room.

"What's the problem, man?"

"Uhh, you didn't give me anything for my cold."

"Wait, wait, wait, I spent ten minutes with you discussing your infected tattoo, and more importantly, what to do about getting an erection going forward. Not once did you mention that you had a cold."

"I forgot. Also, can I get those pills we talked about?"

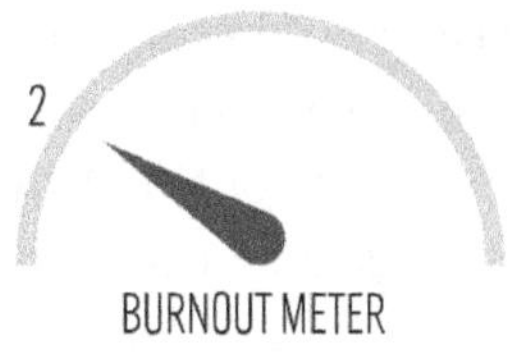

Biloxi Blues

Mississippi, 2005
Hurricane Katrina

From one disaster to another.

Because of my experience as a NYC medic, I was volunteered as the first from my PA class to go to Mississippi after Hurricane Katrina. I had no idea what to expect after being attached to a group of DO professors and med students from Nova Southeastern University (I know, multidirectional schools are not always synonymous with higher learning, but I promise you the training was tough as hell).

We hastily gathered in a dented passenger van for the ride from Ft. Lauderdale to Biloxi and other parts of Mississippi most affected by the hurricane. The briefing would take place en route, but ostensibly, NSU was providing current and future medical professionals to set up clinics, distribute medicine, and deliver food and necessities to displaced hurricane victims. Excited to get out of the classroom. Honored that my pedigree got me assigned to this important mission, back on the front lines.

As we drove through the Florida Panhandle, I heard

whispers in the van about our driver sweating profusely and noticeably shaking as he peered into the oncoming headlights. I guess the doctors and professors made their decision about the risk of DTs vs. driving 800 miles with someone who was legally drunk, because our driver grabbed a sixer at his first opportunity from a restaurant cooler and disappeared back to the van. Instead, I ate disappointing pizza from a joint using a letterboard menu in eastern Alabama (I thought better of sharing this development with my wife, Lori, who was six months pregnant with our first child).

Deep into the second year of my PA program, I had experienced the pros and cons of grad school. During my OB rotation (thankfully no longer mandatory), the nurse midwife, who absolutely hated my guts, told me if I agreed to *not* show up for deliveries in the hospital, she would give me a B. If I didn't show up for the STD clinic, I would get an F. I may have a soft spot for pregnant women, but not so much for gonorrhea. When yet another Florida hurricane got me out of most of my stirrup and swab sessions, I was hardly disappointed.

I also worked at a children's clinic in one of the poorest areas of Ft. Lauderdale with the most appreciative patients I've ever cared for. Nestled between the bowels of the airport and dying jai alai frontons, Haitian families with no insurance, underinsured working class, and anyone with general disdain for most doctors filled the waiting room of this long-established community clinic. Almost every patient encounter seemed meaningful and appreciated. At the end of a rewarding six weeks, the owner extended an open job offer to me.

But my heart belonged to emergency medicine, so I

held out.

As I chatted with the med students (all younger than me) along our Southern adventure, I hoped that this journey landed in the "pro" column. Bonding over hot Waffle House coffee, I was comforted by my real-world experience far outweighing their med-school training. We finally pulled into one of the endless buildings with a rooftop cross near Biloxi. Exhausted and a little disoriented, I was offered a cot in the middle of a Baptist church floor.

Before I could shut my eyes, no less than three parishioners accosted me and asked if I had accepted Jesus Christ as my Lord and Savior.

"That's a NO," from this Cleveland Jew.

The next day, we drove past the beached Grand Casino riverboat barge, marooned in the middle of the highway like a New Wave Ballardian cover. We drove past unnaturally twisted buildings, and trees with lost laundry and bike parts hanging from dead branches. Local businesses with awnings torn and windows shattered. Boarded-up houses with homemade plywood signs that said *Holla at your Girl* and a phone number to let neighbors know they had made it. American spirit on tsunami soil.

A small fishing boat parked itself in the Burger King drive-thru window. Families rummaged in the piles of their lost homes and businesses, more in search of sentiment than value. While it wasn't New Orleans, there was no sense that these towns were any less in need of a little humanity and a lot of help.

Our first priority: establish a pop-up clinic where local residents could receive their life-saving medications. Not provide medical care or triage. While the other students and I organized a makeshift pharmacy inside a still-standing civic center, the doctors set up curtained stations, ready to take quick histories and match meds to patients. A good feeling spread in the group as sleepiness gave way to purpose and anticipation.

Long lines formed at the doors, and patients presented laundry lists of medications. Common diabetes and blood pressure pills like Metformin, Atenolol, and Lasix flew off the shelves as I raced to unpack hospital and pharmacy donations. Plenty of penicillin and Z-Paks, along with piles of allergy meds and steroid creams. Finally, a chance to get back in the field and reap the rewards of a twenty-seven-month-long graduate school life pause was here! All of the mind-numbing PowerPoints slogged through while pretzeled into bolted-down metal chairs. All of the rotations spent doing menial medical tasks for disinterested docs. The expensive tradeoff for graduating from an algorithmic processor of medical emergencies to being able to recall rare endocrine or neurological conditions even twenty years later.

The last time I felt this level of satisfaction was signing off over NYC EMS radio on my last shift. Axler on the mic one last time, to let all of New York know I was moving on from a never-imagined career as a Lenox Hill medic to a higher level of patient care.

That feeling faded before my next Waffle House feeding.

The lines remained long throughout the morning, and the crowd got younger and younger. Requests for medications I wasn't familiar with filtered back to our little pharmacy closet. Lortab, Lorcet, Norco, T3, Roxicet, Tylox . . . but none were on our shelves. It didn't occur to me, and certainly not to the medical directors, that the promise of a "pop-up clinic" with no prior patient charts was an open invitation to every drug seeker in the entire region.

By the third hour, we posted signs that said, *No Oxy/Hydrocodone/Codeine.*

By the fourth hour, the lines disappeared entirely.

As we traveled through Biloxi and Kiln and other small cities across southern Mississippi, we hung signs at the door to start the day. *NO NARCOTICS.* Aside from a little morning push, our clinics were almost empty within an hour. Despite taking care of methadone maintenance zombies and heroin ODs on a regular basis in NYC, nothing prepared me for the OxyContin-induced opioid epidemic that had come.

I had left my pregnant wife for a week to sit in a cramped van with strangers, sleep on church floors, and shit in porta-potties only to be greeted as a drug dealer.

I imagined it would pay better.

The Southern skies were clear and so was I-10. While we dished out one more assembly-line breakfast, the docs hurriedly shoveled remaining meds and supplies into coolers. A return to the realities of school and a kicking baby awaited. A burnt group, more than anxious to tag-in the next wave of volunteers, grabbed their packs and slumped into the van.

The med students allayed any letdown with resume-builder justification.

But I knew this was a fucking failure.

An ominous silence as we rode home. A combination of devastating disappointment and pretend naps to avoid chatter. Any words of false praise about "difference making" from the docs who had clearly given up by Day 3 were met with low groans. And I had 800 miles to go, to think about whether I now had the heart to tell Lori and my classmates that the most important thing I handed out over the entire week was food, not medicine.

I keep a folder of pictures from that trip on a time-warped Kodak CD. A group photo in front of the van, wearing both our school T-shirts and hopeful smiles before the trip began:

Teeth brushed with bottled water.

Children hugging my leg in gratitude.

Laughter around tater-tot breakfasts.

Churches standing unscathed while they sheltered and served the needy.

Sun shining after the storm.

And then darker pictures: cabinets full of unclaimed Tylenol and Motrin. First aid supplies in stacks waiting to dress wounded that never came. The windblown riverboat washed away on tilt, never to be righted again. As washed away as the hope of a new shift whenever I saw an out-of-state van parked at my clinic. A reminder that between heroin and fentanyl, there was legalized opium in the form of OxyContin.

When I left New York, I only knew methadone as heroin maintenance replacement. In Florida, it was popped like Tums for pain management. Fentanyl was used for hospice patients and ketamine was something that people stole from veterinary clinics.

I was both proud of what we had set out to do, and slapped with the disconnect between theory and practice that would haunt the rest of my career.

Like weeds taking hold in a well-intended garden.

But that would still be years away.

I had bigger concerns. Like grabbing another sixer from Dolly's Quick Stop to lube our driver.

And getting home to kiss Lori's belly.

    American Triage

5

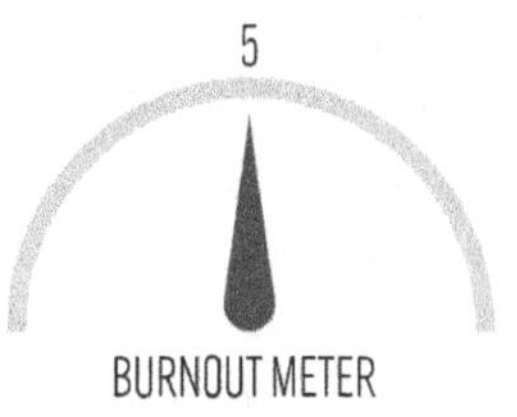

BURNOUT METER

A Little Bit of Knowledge

Palm Beach Gardens, Florida 2010s

"You're not going to believe this!"

"Try me, I've seen some stuff."

"No, you've never seen anything like *this*."

"I can't stand the suspense. Take your sock off."

My forty-something male patient wearing scrubs gingerly rolls his sock down, occasionally pausing for a dramatic wince, to reveal a slightly swollen big toe. Then the rambling begins.

"It's green, doc, my toe is green! I don't know if it's sepsis or a DVT [blood clot], but it's killing me! The pain goes all the way to my carpals [those are in the hand]. I sent a picture to a nurse friend of mine and she said . . ."

Oh my god, make it stop, make it stop . . .

". . . and she said it needs to be lanced immediately."

And that's why I want it to stop. In only a few seconds this patient has told me everything I need to know about why this encounter is going to be a nightmare. Aside from the histrionics of a grown man yelling about his toe, there is a smattering of medical terminology used. This is a patient's subtle way of telling me,

"Hey man, I'm in the club, I know what I'm talking about."

Then there is the reference to a consult with another medical professional, who has already provided my patient with bad information and false expectations.

But this might be his wife, his sister, or his neighbor, so instead of saying "Are you fucking kidding me?" I say, "Slow down, my friend. Let's go back to when you actually hurt yourself. What happened?"

"I kicked a tree."

"You kicked a tree? When?"

"A few hours ago, and now my toe is green!"

"Your toe is not green. You have a boo-boo. That's a little bit of blood collecting under your nail and that is *black*, not green."

What I see is about a half-centimeter sliver of a black line across his toenail that in no way represents a serious injury or a need for burning a hole through his nail to drain the underlying blood. I explain this to him.

"What about antibiotics, what about a DVT!!!!"

"Are you in school?"

"Yes! I'm studying to be a [fill in any medical certificate program here]."

At this point, my brain is fighting to either shut down completely or force a nod. Those two forces arm wrestle and instead what comes out is, "Okay, I need you to stop talking. I don't know what they're teaching you at school, but nothing you're saying is right. This is Ortho 101. You don't get an infection or a blood clot in your leg from stubbing your toe. That's crazy talk. This is ice, rest, and Motrin, simple as that. You don't get antibiotics for a bruise, and you don't develop a clot in your calf four hours after bumping your toe."

Finally my guy does stop talking. A smile returns to his face and he says, "You know what they say about a little bit of knowledge . . ."

Dangerous? Try mind-numbing. It's the same Seinfeldian routine that brings in chiropractors to treat minor aches and pains, or for post-car-accident care.

"Nah, I don't want X-rays."

Seriously?

Your whole profession is built on taking unnecessary X-rays! If I were *your* patient, this would be the first in a series of thousands of X-rays! But when it comes to your own care, you acknowledge it's a waste of time. The same routine that recently prompted a nurse I was treating for a cold to tell me,

"Oh, by the way, I've been having palpitations for six months."

"Where do you work?"

"In cardiac telemetry."

Of course you do. That *beep beep beep* noise? Oh, never mind . . .

A few of the medics from our city's fire department pull shifts at the clinic on off days. **They're great.** And the medics who respond to our occasional 9-1-1 calls for chest pain or stroke-like symptoms know that I'm not wasting their time; these are real emergencies. As a former medic, when one of them comes to the clinic with a family member as a patient, they have all of my attention.

A dad brought his teen son with fever and nausea with sudden onset that morning. He was sure it was food poisoning, but wanted him checked out. After examining the son, who looked toxic, I urged the medic to take him to the

ER for a possible appendicitis. After a brief argument, he agreed to take his son to hospital. I said I hoped that I was wrong, but knew that I wasn't.

When I called him four hours later to check on his son, the appendix was on an operating room tray and the boy was recovering from surgery. When the clinic opened on Monday, he called the manager to request a refund because I "hadn't done anything for him."

You're welcome.

Great Catch

"Pathology is on the phone for you."

"You mean radiology?"

"No, *pathology*, dumbass."

Becca and I had a special PA–Nurse relationship. Orders and workflow were more interpretive than concrete. Her years of ER experience sometimes colliding with my straight-out-of-school overconfidence, before she would go on to become an excellent PA herself.

Pathology? Did we even have a pathology department at this hospital? I was a little confused and certainly *not* confident as I reached for the in-house phone . . .

The attending that day was one of the per diem docs, only occasionally making an appearance to fill a shift and probably at double the normal rate. I always liked this guy. He didn't give a shit about taking orders from the ER manager or telling a specialist to suck it. Once, he overheard an orthopedist berating me over the phone about the specific angulation of a fractured tibia. Aware that I was getting chewed out, he grabbed the phone out of my hands.

"Listen! The bone is broken in twenty-eight fucking places and we don't have a protractor. Get down here, reduce it yourself, and do your fucking job."

He calmly handed the phone back to me.

"All set."

So I was at ease as we stretched into the afternoon, clearing rooms quickly in Fast Track, when a man in his thirties disappeared behind a curtain with his family in tow. Becca slipped back into our work nook and handed me a chart with perfectly normal vitals that had been triaged only as "headache."

I pulled back the curtain to find my patient holding hands with his concerned wife, and two braided-hair little girls, barely older than my daughters, climbing all over their dad like a new toy.

"Hi, guys. I'm Adam and I'm going to help you today."

My patient was dressed in one of those short sleeve button-ups with a permanent oval name tag sewn in. One that let you know he worked a hard job, worked with his hands for a living. Even though he had clearly come straight from work, his shirt was clean and pressed. A sign of self-respect and respect for us at the hospital.

As he looked nervously towards his wife, she got the conversation started.

"He's been having headaches for three months now. Today, it got worse."

"Ehh, it's nothing. She made me come."

"When did the headaches start (was it really three months)?" I asked. His chart didn't indicate a history of headaches or sickle cell disease. I kept probing.

"What do they feel like? Are they always at the same time of day? How long do they last?

   American Triage

"Nah, she's exaggerating. I just pop an aspirin or two and that usually works."

"Tell the doctor the truth," his wife insisted. "You told me you could barely see today!"

While I appreciated the upgrade from PA to MD (again, respectful), I was getting concerned. This guy wasn't going to complain about anything, and sure as hell wasn't going to look up a local neurologist on his day off.

"I'm going to order a few tests. We're going to draw your blood and get a CAT scan of your head. It's like getting a picture of your brain. Let's see if we can get some answers."

Both he and his wife thanked me, and the girls shouted "**THANK YOU**" in unison as I left the makeshift ER room.

I entered orders into the computer and got back to my other patients. Casting a wide net, hoping for a CT *without* a softball-sized tumor and a simple neuro referral. I nodded in passing to the rad tech as he wheeled my guy down the hall.

After discharging a few easy cases and allowing myself five minutes of solitude in the breakroom, I returned to my station.

"Pathology is on the phone for you."

Getting a call from a specialist was never good news. Even at this early stage in my career, I knew it meant one of only three things:

I fucked up.

The specialist wanted more testing to cover their ass.

Or worse, *neither.*

I refreshed the test results on my screen as I sat down.

CT Brain Without Contrast: Negative.

Lab results: only one number in red. *150.*

I reached for the receiver.

"Hi, this is the PA."

"Hello, this Dr. (whoever). Umm, uh, I'm calling because your patient has a WBC (white blood cell count, the ones that fight infection) of *150 thousand.* I recommend that he be admitted for further testing, but this number is consistent with some sort of leukemia."

Click.

Fuck.

I was no pathologist, but I knew a normal white count was around 10,000. I scrolled down the on-call list and dialed the hospitalist.

"150,000?" They agreed to admit and consult oncology immediately.

I slinked by the half-open curtain on my way to tell the attending the bad news. My patient was now back in his room, two loving girls in his stretcher laying against his hospital gown.

"What made you think to order labs on a headache patient?" the attending said.

"I didn't like the story. I didn't like any of it."

"That's a great catch!"

I was momentarily flattered by the praise. When I look back though, that flattery is in doubt. Was his enthusiasm out of mutual respect, for sifting through the routine ER noise? Or was it because this new PA saved him from a missed leukemia diagnosis on his watch, saved him from a lawsuit? Was the gauge on *his* burnout meter at seven already? Long past the thought of "damn, this guy has cancer," to only, "hmm, that's an interesting case."

"Yeah, great fucking catch," I said. "I get to be the first person to tell him, in front of his family, that he's going to

die."

The Timeline: Part 2

1028:

BOOM!

Fuck. Steve? Run!

The towers don't collapse like a toddler knocking over an architecturally flawed Lego creation. They sink, like pulling the wrong Jenga piece from the bottom few rows. Like the devil smashing pancake stacks on top of each other. The smells of diesel and Manhattan summer heat, my own fresh sweat, dissipate as the North Tower projectile vomits down Vesey Street.

We are way too close, but we don't freeze.

No matter what happens, stay together, stay alive.

We run.

And run.

While we can still see the silhouettes of humans and cars, over broken pavement.

Then, *the cloud.*

Easily enveloping us and distorting survival probabilities. My nose and eyes burn with toxic ash. My throat gargles sour smoke . . . We are smacked with a sonic wave and the dirtiest dust mixture ever compounded.

Infinite sound.

Total blindness.

The snowing ash that covers me and my bus and the

living and the dead. That covers lower Manhattan with chaos. I drop my radio but can still hear the Nextel (which never stops working) beeping.

We are approaching our bus.

I am alive.

Steve is alive.

1030–1032:

Sweat seeps through our BDUs, as the smog of collapsed tower coats the streets, but is still faint enough for us to find our bus. We somehow grab our friend and coworker Jason, running blindly, who has left 11 Young or 10 Charlie abandoned.

Triage?

Not yet.

Survive.

An FDNY firefighter stumbles past in search of his crew, while a dust-drenched survivor running in crazed shock knocks Jason over. I open the passenger door and yank him onto my lap.

"My wife is dead, my wife is dead!"

Screaming, sobbing, I half-hold this stranger in empathy, half for stability. Jason is at the edge of the passenger compartment bench, shaken but wired. Nobody has to tell Steve what to do.

Reverse.

On a good day, visibility in the modified van known as 10 Frank is total shit. Jason shouts out instructions from the rear as Steve navigates a maze of humans, emergency vehicles, and unrelenting adrenaline, *backwards.* We drive to a semblance of a clearing and safety as dust rains over Vesey Street. Bruised skyscrapers linger above, blown-out glass and stalled cruisers below. Glimpses of flashing fire

     American Triage

engines line now-blacked-out streets.

I don't remember what words I speak to the man on my lap. Hopefully, I say something intelligible and human before he escapes aimlessly, releasing from the front seat in a dark panic. Devastated for him, but secretly happy that at least, he's alive.

I never see him again.

We pop open the rear doors and stab holes into saline bottles. I realize I can barely see through fried, dust-caked eyes, so I flush them as best I can.

Only occasionally checking on each other, Steve and I work more like offensive linemen who know how to pass block. Each functioning independently, but completely in tune. We hang IV bags from hooks, grabbing every bottle and bandage we have, and we're open for business like some sort of Faustian food truck.

Firefighters and police officers rush over for eye flushes and bleeding control before disappearing back into their own hells. Civilians are a different story. The ambulance is an oasis, a place to stop and be reassured they are still alive. Each story more horrific than the next, but truthfully, they wash over me while I instinctively pat and scan for unseen wounds.

Is anything broken?
Can I stop the bleeding?
Are you in shock?
Can you walk?
"NEXT!"
Triage. Triage. Triage.
But there are so many . . .

1050:

Limping in circles and muttering curse words, a white-shirted FDNY LT catches our attention near the bus. He hobbles up and down an uneven pile of broken concrete and cinder in hysterical loops, oblivious to his pain and waving us off repeatedly. Steve guides him to rest on the bumper of the ambulance, his ankle clearly broken. Unclear how he made it this far, we gather he has witnessed his friends, his men, die. Another image that haunts me. He allows a simple ace wrap before storming off.

Pure shock.

1105–1119:

Still wired but finally feeling useful, we continue to help everyone we can. Our supplies diminish. The world narrows to the funnel of patients we can treat, or reasonably direct to the Borough of Manhattan Community College gym for further instruction. Steve's functioning radio instructs us to move to St. Vinny's, a few blocks away.

Before we can even settle in to recalibrate, more panic. Navy blue ATF jackets and flashing lights pass us, armed with knowledge we don't have access to.

"Get out of here!"

But where to? Chelsea Piers? What the fuck is going on?

1130–1134:

Connecticut plates. Jersey plates. A *green* fucking ambulance chokes the line! Can you please get out of our goddamn way! Insulted and already battered, the only other medics we want to see are New Yorkers. Our friends from Cornell and Roosevelt and FDNY. The ones who have just gone through it. Are we going to be sent back to the daily grind while buffs from volunteer departments work the towers?

Bullshit.

Steve kind of half-parks, half-angles out in case we need to boogie. It's strange now to think of being staged three miles from Ground Zero. But after being evacuated a second or third time that day to the Piers, *all of NYC feels like Ground Zero.* The thought of being stuck on a collapsing pier and falling into the Hudson River isn't that appealing. The airwaves echo the screams of desperate medics, intermittently cut off by dispatch with conflicting updates. This is the beginning of the threats; anthrax and suspicious packages.

We worry every decision we make might be our last.

Right on cue, dispatch advises us not to park over grates or manhole covers.

Bomb.

Rumors and panic run rampant. One of our New York unit buddies tells us another plane has crashed, this one near Pittsburgh.

Pittsburgh?

My world is no longer narrow and small. It is gaping open.

Lori.

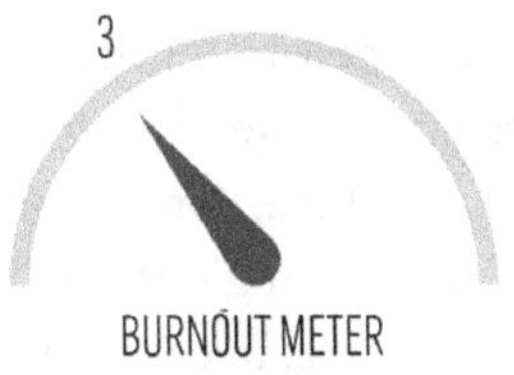

Batteries Not Included

Port St. Lucie ER, Florida 2007

Swamped with sutures, MVAs (motor vehicle accidents), and nebulous belly pains, I was rarely called over to the main ER from the Fast Track area in the middle of a shift. But something stunk, and this had the makings of a shit-runs-downhill-from-the-doc-to-the-PA kind of case. Behind a patient curtain near the ambulance bay, a whimpering middle-aged man lay prone with his ass barely covered by a too-small hospital gown. Shrinking in the corner, a woman.

Not his wife.

Much can get lost in the interpretation of a pre-coded medical form under the heading of *FOREIGN BODY.* For example, sometimes it's a Crayola lodged up a child's nose. Sometimes it's a tampon a patient couldn't remember removing. A snapped Q-tip end stuck inside an ear canal (very satisfying to retrieve).

And sometimes, it's a sordid midweek affair, a failed safe word, and eventually, a vibrator. I stepped outside the curtain and after a few brief words with the doc, understood that this guy wasn't the only one being screwed. I ordered a sedative, returned to my station to discharge a few patients, and prepared to get dirty.

Armed with surgical lube, forceps that could flip bacon from five feet away, rubber gloves (no need for sterility where I was going) and a mask in case of blowback, I pulled up a stool to the edge of the stretcher. In PA school, we had paid volunteers come in for a few awkward evenings spent learning how to perform vaginal and prostate exams. But there was no *asshole foreign body removal* practicum or corresponding lecture. I was on my own.

Aside from the pressure of performing the procedure for an audience, two other distracting forces were at play. First, the series of "what the fuck are we going to tell our spouses" whispers. Second, my inner monologue of wheezing laughter and absurdity of the situation. I bit my tongue and suddenly appreciated Seinfeld's dilemma of going to see *Plan 9 From Outer Space* alone. What was I going to do, make sarcastic remarks to myself?

I allowed time for the Ativan to kick in, or at least, tamper the screams from each probe of a finger or forceps. Every minute or two, a nurse would pop a head in to offer assistance, but truthfully, they came out of morbid curiosity and as an excuse to tell the story firsthand after their shift. Progress slowed as my hand cramped inside this man's butt. Maybe Ortho or Derm would've been a better career choice.

But I'm a professional, and foreign-body removals can be damn satisfying cases. Fish hooks meant for Mahi, roofing nails through feet, pasta under fingernails, wineglass stems, splinters, BBs, and cockroaches. So I blocked out the groans as my forceps probed for something to grab on to, and got to work.

Slowly and deliberately, progress was being made. My forceps caught the edge of something. I kept pinching the edge with a gentle tug. Over and over, despite my patient's protests, I reached back for the prize like a naive child operating the claw machine at a rigged arcade. There was resistance, release, and the hope of success. Wishing Loretta Swit was wiping the sweat off my forehead, I went back in.

Yes!

I had removed something.

But there was a problem.

What I had between the prongs of my forceps was not a two-dollar teddy bear, but the phallus's end cap. The bulk of the vibrator still lost in a dark hole. Unlike the satisfaction of opening a pickle jar after a long struggle, the vice grip from this guy's colon had only succeeded in allowing me to twist, not pull. And while the funmaker runs on batteries, people do not. I was now at risk of having them slide out into his anal cavity. Leaving Duracells inside a human body is not a good thing.

Imagine the Customer Service Survey.

Time to punt this fucker.

Disgusted, I disposed of my blood-and-shit-stained gloves, washed my hands, and stormed over to a phone to summon an unsuspecting on-call surgeon. The ER doctor predictably asked me, "How are things going in there?" I muttered words like "vibrator," "stuck," and "batteries" into the phone before slamming it down. Like Snake Doctor from *The Unit* said, "Once in, never out!"[13]

---

[13] *The Unit*, created by Shawn Ryan, aired on CBS, 2006–2009.

The (Jenny) McCarthyism of Modern Medicine

United Kingdom 2000s or United States now

Americans more likely to take medical advice from Playboy Bunny than Surgeon General or CDC.

It sounds like a bad joke, and it would be if it weren't true. Not only did Jenny McCarthy, a former *Playboy* centerfold, blame vaccines as the cause for her son's autism, but she would later claim his autism was "cured" through a combination of diet and chelation therapy. "The University of Google," she told Oprah, "is where I got my degree from."[14]

But every few weeks I have a patient encounter with a panicked parent that goes something like this:

"I think my son has the mumps!"

"It's not possible."

---

[14] Katrina vanden Heuvel, "Jenny McCarthy's Vaccination Fear-Mongering and the Cult of False Equivalence," *The Nation*, July 22, 2013, https://www.thenation.com/article/archive/jenny-mccarthys-vaccination-fear-mongering-and-cult-false-equivalence/.

"But I looked it up on WebMD."

"No, I mean, it's not possible because we *vaccinate* for mumps."

"Oh, well I, I mean we . . ."

"You what . . . ?"

"We don't believe in vaccinations. I'm a spiritualist."

Funny how many of these spiritualists/McCarthyites lose their spirit when it comes to whisking their kids in for unnecessary antibiotics, their willingness to put their ten-year-olds on multiple behavior meds, or requesting benzodiazepines for themselves. The hypocrisy is enormous.

"Hmm, did you call your pediatrician?"

"Well . . ."

"Oh, I'm sorry, silly question. You don't have a pediatrician because no pediatrician in their right mind would allow you in their practice without vaccinating your child against dangerous communicable diseases. It's too big a liability for themselves and their other, compliant patients. But you thought you'd pop into your local urgent care and be evaluated for a possible illness that only an infectious disease doctor or pediatric specialist has ever seen. Never mind exposing *our* elderly and pediatric patients to your child."

Things tend to get a little uncomfortable after that, but I proceed with the history and exam. Even though the child is inevitably afflicted with a routine viral sore throat or exanthem (rash), the parent soon asks for "mumps testing."

"We don't test for mumps."

"What do we do if it is mumps?"

"I don't know, perhaps acquire a time machine and head back a few years to that day you decided to not vaccinate your child with the hopes that nothing bad would ever hap-

pen and simultaneously count on the herd immunity provided by responsible parents who did."

"I'm serious! What if it is mumps, can something bad
happen?"

"Oh, other than your child ending up in the hospital
with IVs hanging from both arms because he can't swallow,
deafness, meningitis, or infertility with horrible testicular
pain, no, nothing bad can happen. By the way, what school
does he go to?"

"Why?"

"Because if it's the same school as my child, I want to
inform the principal that you're not allowed back until
cleared by a specialist."

Despite the fact that Andrew Wakefield, the original author of a whopping twelve (yes, twelve)-patient retro-
spective study attempting to link autism to the use of the
MMR (measles, mumps, rubella) vaccine, is now banned
from practicing medicine ever again, despite the fact that
he was found guilty of thirty-six counts of fraud, parents
still fall back upon his research. The British, armed with
this study that wouldn't pass standards for a fifth-grade
science project, embarked on an anti-vaccination campaign. Guess what happened?

Based on this bogus study, the United Kingdom and
Ireland stopped vaccinating en masse. Parts of London
had vaccination rates as low as *61*% in 2003, far below the
rate needed to avoid an epidemic of measles.[15] The effects
weren't seen immediately, as it took a few years for these
unvaccinated infants to grow up. But by 2005, the UK had

---

[15] Simon Murch, "Separating Inflammation From Speculation in Autism," *The Lancet* 362, no. 9394 (November 1, 2003): 1498–99, https://
doi.org/10.1016/s0140-6736(03)14699-5.

its first measles death in almost fifteen years, and in the first month of 2006, *5000* cases of mumps were reported, epidemic proportions.

The European McCarthyites, long able to hide behind Wakefield's bogus study and responsible parents and pediatricians, were no longer safe themselves. Herd immunity was gone. The same type of parent shows up at my clinic with a health-department form asking for a "religious exemption," expecting me to allow their unvaccinated child to hide out among "the herd." No fucking way, but good luck with homeschool (there are a lot of homeschoolers in my state). And now the joke is on me as our surgeon general is eliminating vaccination requirements *entirely*.

In 2004, Wakefield's study was only partially retracted by *The Lancet*, not to be fully rescinded until 2010, long after the damage had been done. The MMR vaccination-autism scare has been called "the most damaging medical hoax of the last 100 years."[16]

But as the CDC is being dismantled by an anti-vax former heroin addict, the hoax persists.

Despite their holy grail of evidence being shredded as *National Enquirer* type fodder, McCarthy is only the tip of this sinking iceberg. The concept of spurious correlation doesn't exist for these people. Study after study also demonstrates the omission bias exhibited by parents. When presented with evidence that *not* vaccinating their child will cause them to die at a rate of 10:10,000 versus the vaccine itself directly causing death at a rate of, say,

---

[16] Dennis K Flaherty, "The Vaccine-Autism Connection: A Public Health Crisis Caused by Unethical Medical Practices and Fraudulent Science," *Annals of Pharmacotherapy* 45, no. 10 (September 13, 2011): 1302–4, https://doi.org/10.1345/aph.1q318.

5:10,000, many still choose not to vaccinate.[17] Uh, this is *doubling* your child's chances of death!

A new Danish study of over *one million* children shows there is no link between vaccinations and autism. Or fifty other chronic disorders including asthma and ADHD.[18] Instead, scientists have established a link between vaccinations and preventing the communicable diseases that they vaccinate for.

Dr. Jake Scott, infectious disease specialist and professor at the Stanford University School of Medicine, stated, "Vaccines have been the most thoroughly vetted of all medicines. Not only are the safety profiles being studied during the trials, they're also being monitored after licensure like nothing else. I mean, we have so much more safety data on vaccines than we do on supplements, which a lot of people have no issue taking [thanks for the bonus jab at pseudoscience!]."[19]

Ever heard of polio? Perhaps not, because due to a vigilant vaccination campaign, polio was eradicated in this country in 1979. However, during the 1940s and 1950s poliomyelitis crippled thousands of patients. Polio can lead to permanent paralysis and death. Something you would

---

[17] Ilana Ritov and Jonathan Baron, "Reluctance to Vaccinate: Omission Bias and Ambiguity," *Journal of Behavioral Decision Making* 3, no. 4 (October/December 1990): 263–77, https://doi.org/10.1002/bdm.3960030404.

[18] Niklas Worm Andersson et al., "Aluminum-Adsorbed Vaccines and Chronic Diseases in Childhood," *Annals of Internal Medicine*, July 15, 2025, https://doi.org/10.7326/annals-25-00997.

[19] Chris Dall, "Vaccine RCT Spreadsheet Aims to Show the Data, Dispel Myths About Vaccines," *CIDRAP*, June 18, 2025, https://www.cidrap.umn.edu/adult-non-flu-vaccines/vaccine-rct-spreadsheet-aims-show-data-dispel-myths-about-vaccines.

think most parents would want to avoid. Whole summers were lost. Parents were mortified to let their kids leave the house. You were negligent, an outcast, if you weren't lined up for the vaccine.

But the pendulum has swung!

In light of the politicization of vaccinations during COVID, long-established vaccines have come under question and we are in line for a UK-style herd immunity failure over the next ten years (measles is already here!). So when your patients and neighbors start talking about vaccine-induced autism with a straight face, it's hard to not blow a gasket.

There is no debate.

There is no discussion.

There is no evidence!

How do you argue with that? You can't. You only wish the best for their children and hope that they decide to homeschool or better yet, move.

There Will Be Signs

Palm Beach Gardens, Florida 2016

I'm still heartbroken that medicine let me down, but I saw the writing on the wall long before I quit. Not-so-subtle hints that let me know I was more a blackjack dealer dressed in scrubs than a scientist put into place to actually help people.

As a PA working eighteen twelve-hour shifts per month, I asked management for a new chair to replace my increasingly broken one. After a few weeks of sending fruitless messages, I finally received an email from the regional manager asking me to fill out ADA (Americans with Disabilities Act) paperwork to justify my request. The same manager who had asked me a dozen times to call in meds for her and her family. In return, she sent me a link to a form.

My hopes sank as quickly as my chair's failing hydraulics. An involuntary "fuck" escaped into the communal work space, a hedged-in square with no privacy for docs or nurses. Gossip of my coworkers also getting screwed quickly circulated after detailing my inane email.

I rolled my shitty chair down the hall past my coworkers, outside, and then over the cobbled brick walkway two doors down to where our unattached kitchen and breakroom were. Also inside was the posh office of the clinic's seldomly seen owner. Long checked out, he would only pop in to inform us of the millions waiting for him upon a corporate buyout. Counting the days until he never had to practice medicine again.

A true inspiration.

Behind the French doors, he kept a wine-storage cabinet, an oversized desk, and his spare clubs. And, where he also kept a throne-sized leather chair complete with functioning levers.

Resisting the urge to put a new driver through an old Bordeaux, I dumped my Office Depot clunker and wheeled my new ride outside. Ignoring the applause and hysterical cackling of my coworkers, I pretended to stoically resume work. The giggling became too hard to control as I spun around like a child, before offering free rides to all. Everyone took a turn, cruising to X-ray, or lounging and reclining in complete comfort for a change. Full-on Bond and Austin Powers villain reenactments ensued. A medic sank back and took a nap during his hour in the new seat.

King for a day.

My chair was back by the next shift.

Despite my urgent care being purchased by a United-Healthcare subsidiary (yes the same company whose CEO was murdered), employees were not offered any sort of UHC plan, let alone any discounted healthcare. The reason given was that they did not want to upset their Blue Cross Blue Shield contracted centers in Pennsylvania. When I started as a paramedic at Lenox Hill Hospital in

2000, my health insurance was *free*, and when I added Lori it was fourteen dollars per month.

Speaking of Lenox Hill, I once got a call from my supervisor at seven in the morning, right before I left for my shift.

"Don't come in today. You're off until next week."

Fearful that I had done something wrong, I eked out a *"Why not?"* But this old-school medic wasn't busting my balls. He was watching my back.

"You've accrued too much sick time; if you don't use it, you'll lose it."

Too much sick time? I'm still laughing, thinking about it. In my subsequent twenty years in medicine, I took exactly **ZERO** sick days. Once, I even handed my jury duty summons to my ER manager and he threw it in the trash like I had personally stolen money from him. A job where I was exposed to flu, strep, pneumonia, and a seasonal smorgasbord of viral illnesses on a daily basis, and management didn't allow for their own employees to get sick. Or to perform my civic duty.

Medicine is full of acronyms. EKG, CPR, IV; but apparently COLA isn't one of them. Justification for a fifty-two-cent raise one year was that I could "easily be replaced" by a nurse practitioner for less money, so I should be thankful for anything I got. I'm not even sure how you arrive at a figure so small as to be intentionally insulting, but no, I was not thankful.

There was a tipping point not that long ago when science almost won. Hordes of academic papers about using antibiotics sparingly, Presidents Bush and Obama preparing for Bird Flu and Ebola outbreaks. And now, back to bleach and measles. Fear about long-term issues with medicine now looks prescient with RFK Jr., Secretary of Human and Health Services, saying, "I don't think people should be taking medical advice from me."

Unreal.

A multitude of factors have been working against PA advancement for years, not the least of which has been our own ineptitude. Too complacent about a perceived symbiotic relationship with doctors as the golden children of physician extension, about the only thing we accomplished as a group over the last twenty years was debating whether or not Physician Associate sounded classier than Physician Assistant.

Who gives a fuck!

In the meantime nursing has much better lobbyists, and while they have been able to gain autonomy for practitioners, PAs, especially in states like Florida, remain in the Dark Ages. The only way to make more money is to work more hours. I jumped jobs several times in hopes of finding the right balance. My last serious interview was with a hair transplant specialist. I asked for a percentage of profits from procedures in otherwise vacant surgical suites. His counter was a 20% pay cut plus a two-hour daily commute from my urgent care job.

I was in my car, pretending to be on dinner break, when the office manager delivered this insulting offer with a pride not used to rejection.

"So, less money, more hours than I'm working now?"

"Yes, but you get to train with the great . . ."

Click.

Instead of celebrating my ticket out of urgent care, I started pulling my hair out in the parking lot.

Damn.

I might need those grafts soon. And I was hoping for

a discount.

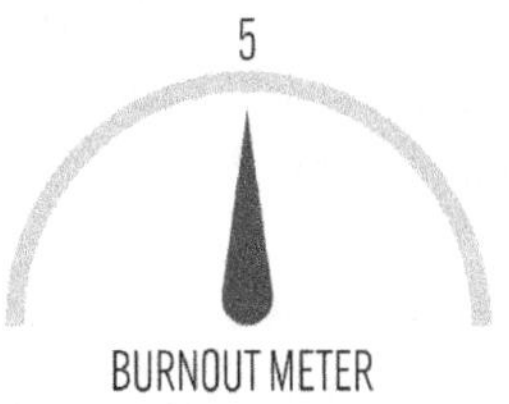

Case Study: I'm Tweaking Brah

Definitely Royal Palm Beach, Florida 2014ish

It's never a good sign when a forty-year-old man wearing a pizza delivery boy shirt with clown-colored shorts hanging halfway down his legs is waiting in the exam room.

"Hi, what brings you in today?"

"Doc, I cut the inside of my ear against the side of my nightstand getting out of bed this morning. It really hurts."

Cool story, except for that being a physical impossibility. That's when I started taking in the whole picture. Dilated pupils, sweaty and greasy, aged beyond his years, and scratches and abrasions all over his arms, neck, and face.

There is an agitation that shouldn't be there. I'm trying to talk to him, but he's all over the map and he keeps scratching himself and scratching and scratching. Finally, I say, "Dude, you have to stop, it's driving me nuts."

The picture becomes clearer. What teeth he has left are mostly yellow and pitted. He reeks of cigarettes and rotting breath, but I decide to go with it.

"So, you have a little scratch in your ear," I say as I retract the otoscope and discard the speculum in the hazardous waste bin. I stroll over to the drawer and immediately clean my scope with an alcohol pad, only to turn around and find brah with a finger in his ear.

"Doc . . ."

"Dude, take your finger out of your ear."

"Sorry, doc [immediately replaces finger back in ear]. Uh, like, if there's any way you can keep me from making pizzas for a few days . . ."

"What the hell are you talking about?"

"Well, you know, how am I gonna flip the pizzas and everything; I don't want to get flour in my ear. The flour goes all over the place [continues to scratch incessantly]."

"Dude, dude! *Stop it!* You cannot scratch your ear or it will start bleeding again, you cannot put a Q-tip in your ear, you cannot put a washcloth in your ear. You have to leave it alone. I'm going to give you drops to make it feel better, but you have to leave it alone."

Not two minutes later I'm back with his prescription and discharge papers, and he's rifling through my drawers. Sure, he's grabbing bandages and gauze but lo and behold, he's also got a Q-tip in his hand.

"*What the fuck are you doing?* Not only are you stealing from me but you're doing the one thing I explicitly asked you not to do, putting a Q-tip in your ear!"

"Sorry man, I'm sorry, I'm sorry, I'm sorry, I didn't mean to steal from you," but he continues to scratch and itch and scratch and itch. He grabs a paper towel from the sink and puts it right in his ear. This is what we call tweaking and this is when I asked him to get out of my clinic as soon as possible.

Damn you, crystal meth! I loved that pizza place!

Kakonomics

Urgent Care USA, Past 2 Decades

Perhaps this is what disgusts Taleb (see "Antiscience") when he refers to the fragile. Easy access to medical care and medications can sometimes do more harm than good. But the negotiations that take place between patient and provider can take another insidious form.

Kakonomics.

Kakonomics refers to the preference for the suboptimal exchange of goods or outcomes between two parties. This theory was put forth by Italian philosopher Gloria Origgi, who tried to put into perspective our universal acceptance of the mediocre.[20] How can this be when it would seem to be human nature to try to optimize every transaction?

This occurs in almost any patient encounter I have throughout the day. Writing an antibiotic for a viral or an

---

[20] Gloria Origgi, "Kakonomics, or the strange preference for Low-quality outcomes," 2011, https://gloriaoriggi.blogspot.com/2011/01/kakonomics-or-strange-preference-for.html

allergic process is a suboptimal solution (useless actually), but it satiates the desire of patients for immediate relief. I am agreeing to exchange this benefit for the false belief that I am providing a faster solution than they could otherwise receive by doing nothing. We are coconspirators in the charade that makes urgent care medicine possible. It is a mediocre solution; limited potential benefit for the patient, and the poor practice of medicine on our end.

In return, we get paid and you walk out with your bauble.

Without getting into the more technical details behind game theory, my young daughters asked me what I was writing about in between bites of their lunch. I explained to them that instead of paying $2 for the canned pumpkin I put in their favorite pancakes, I pay $1 for the store brand because we can't tell the difference. But I asked them if it would be worth paying $1 less if that same can was rotten, even if the store pretended it was as good as the other brand.

"No, that's gross, who would do that?"

"If you pay for medication you don't need, to pretend that it might help you feel better, is that any different?"

"That's dumb, Dad."

Oh well, at least someone gets it.

Recently, I took care of a teenage boy who had been coughing for a few weeks. He couldn't have looked healthier, was completely disinterested in the exam, and continuously chatted with his dad without any sign of illness. Upon discharge, I began my stump-speech explanation of how despite no evidence of bacterial infection, an antibiotic prescription that should be held, *not filled* for another few days, would be offered in case the cough persists.

This is when his father felt the need to look up from his iPhone.

"My wife and I are both physicians."

That's great! And what is your fucking point?

"So, do you think it's bacterial, or is it just a virus?" doctor dad says.

"I'm sorry, you're a doctor?"

This is what I said, but here's what I was thinking. You and your wife, with a combined twenty years of medical training, decide to bring your son not to his pediatrician, but to the urgent care, so that we may weigh in on whether or not a mild cough is bacterial? What the hell is wrong with you!

"Yes, but I don't do this kind of medicine."

"Well," I say, "even so, as a doctor, I'm sure you're aware that a mild persistent cough, even if slightly productive, can come from a viral source."

"Yeah, most of the stuff I see like this is viral, but my wife, The Doctor, is worried about the cough."

Weeee Heee! Now we're getting somewhere. Not only are we in the game for a kakonomic arrangement on the medical front, but this guy is removing himself and his wife from their parenting obligations by pretending, at least for these five minutes, that they have no medical knowledge at all. Classy!

"The antibiotic I wrote for your child is primary treatment for both bacterial pneumonia and bronchitis in his age group. So we are covered there if that is your concern. Again, *as a doctor*, I'm sure you're aware that we have no definitive way of establishing a bacterial source in this environment."

"Do you think that *the real doctor* [ouch] might have more insight into whether or not it's bacterial?"

More insight into your son's cold? More insight than the decades of literature readily available to you? More insight into why, as a doctor, you failed to bring your son to his pediatrician?

"I don't know if he will, but I'll be happy to send him in [and he will be thrilled]."

Two minutes later . . .

"What happened?" I say to my doc.

"I told him the same thing you did and he's going to take the antibiotic."

Good to know I'm making a difference.

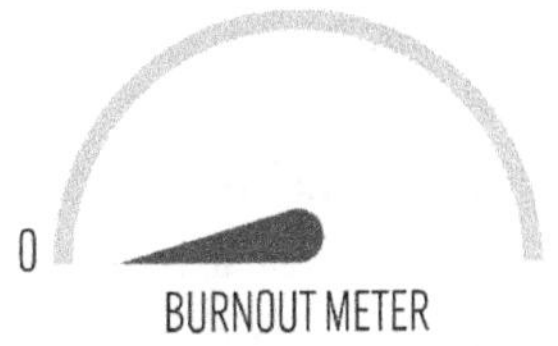

Shit Beer

New York City, 2003

"Open the door!!"

First PD, and now Fire, banging with all their might. I hang back in the hallway, knowing that smell.

Her neighbor called 9-1-1. Hadn't seen her in a few days or heard the TV. And that smell . . .

FD finally says fuck it and brings axe to door. Cheap wood splinters and the hinge cracks, but the door won't budge. Some unknown weight bears against it, and it takes three of us pushing to finally create an opening. One more shove.

At first, a few metallic clinks. An avalanche of Schlitz and shit beer greets us. Piled to the ceiling, tumbling into the hallway like a hailstorm of sour aluminum.

The smell is *outrageous*. Unchanged litter boxes combined with rotting food and vomit.

No life-forms are visible, aside from a few cachectic cats. We wade through the cans, through twenty-year-old *New York Post*s and empty bottles of pure gut-rot whiskey. The small kitchen off to the right is equal parts cat piss and cockroach motel. A police officer pukes in the hallway, too late to cover his nose and mouth.

My partner checks the bathroom. A murky, unflushed bowl and more cat piss. The lone bedroom isn't much better. Unchanged sheets full of ash and shit stains. I check under the bed, inside the accordion closet doors. Nobody home.

We meet in the corridor, more than happy to get the hell out of here, when I spot her.

Like some sort of ancient inebriated elf, pieces of tiny arm and leg poke through Empty Beer Mountain behind the front door. I race over to clear cans from her face and torso, while my partner digs out her legs. Green, vomitous bile suctions her mouth to the door.

Pale and shriveled, she can't weigh more than eighty pounds. I reach for the carotid and apply gentle pressure.

"COCKSUCKER MOTHERFUCKER!!!"

The elf awakens, and aside from being a fan of *The Usual Suspects*, she is super pissed. We jump back, in time to avoid being puked on, but her expletive-filled wrath is only getting started. We try to lift her to the stretcher, but the back of her head is matted to the door with dried blood and . . .

A wig.

I think?

It's glued on at a strange angle, leaving gray wisps protruding over her sunken skull. Snipping into the cartoonishly oversized black hair, my shears free her from the door and we're able to get her loaded on the stretcher.

"GET ME A FUCKING BEER, YOU FUCK-ING ASSHOLES!"

She bucks and hisses against the strain of four men, possessed with shocking effort. But this exorcism will have

American Triage

to take place in the ER. The smell . . .

My partner agrees to drive at dangerous speeds if I agree to sit in the back with the patient and PD.

I grab a mask, place one on her as well.

The officer pukes again before grabbing his mask. We are en route.

"YOUR MOTHER IS A WHORE!"

Soothing sounds as I inflate the blood pressure cuff. Check a radial pulse. Her vital signs? *Not bad.*

BP 98/72, pulse a little tachy at 115. But for someone I assumed was dead ten minutes ago, I'll take it. She is an evil alchemist, apparently capable of converting alcohol into fuel. And curse words.

I search for a semblance of a vein to start an IV, and as I insert the needle . . .

"DIE YOU FUCKING DICK!"

We finally pull into the ER and I can't get the bus doors open fast enough. A little vomit trickles into my mask and I throw it in a red hazard bag, missing its protection immediately.

I give report to the nurse and ER doc, never happier to transfer a patient.

Then the fun starts.

"OWWW. FUCKERS. BEER!!!"

The nurse grabs an emesis basin, saline, and an unlimited supply of gauze. She starts scrubbing.

"BITCH!"

And scrubbing. Dirt and feces ingrained like a tattoo. Caked vomit and fingernails full of black. And the wig.

"FUCKING BITCH!"

The nurse is a pro, but her resolve is waning. Reaching over the old lady's head to clean her back, all the saline has loosened the glue around her scalp. The wig slides off in one giant peel, like a ripped off baseball cover. It reveals scattered open wounds, which drip pus over the nurse's outstretched arms.

It's too much.

The nurse runs over to the sink and heaves violently.

Not once or twice.

Endlessly.

The doc and a few other nurses try to comfort her, but there's no chance. She throws her work badge and gloves into the sink along with her scrub top and announces, "I quit!"

On the way out, she gives the elf the finger.

But before she can clear the sliding doors, we hear:
"GET ME A FUCKING BEER!"

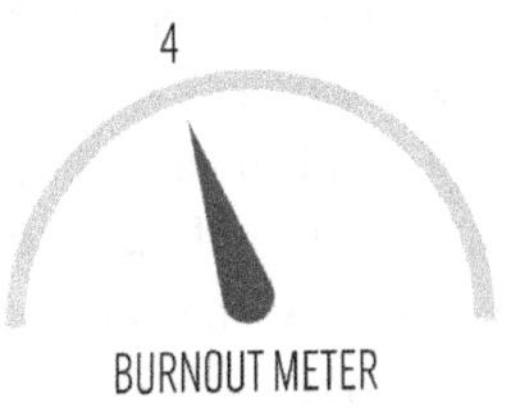

No Good Deed

Boynton Beach, Florida 2011

One of the things I like best about emergency medicine is the shift work. When my day is done, it's done. No paperwork to take home, no overnights on call (standby coverage for a doctor's after-hour service), and not much follow-up. If I can't fix you today, then it's off to the orthopedist, the ENT, or your primary care doctor. But it also puts me in a position to see unique and involved cases due to the sheer volume of high-acuity patients I take care of. Medical curiosity gets the best of me sometimes, and in rare moments of downtime on shift, I'll pick up the phone.

Big mistake.

Crossbow

I recently took care of a teenage girl who thought it might be fun to shoot her boyfriend's high-powered crossbow without any prior training. She left her thumb in the way of the string and came to me with the distal third of her finger hanging sideways with multiple bone fractures. This type of injury is called an "open fracture" because the bone is essentially exposed, and carries a much greater risk of infection and soft-tissue damage.

She was likely a surgical candidate. I performed a digital block, numbing her thumb with lidocaine to provide pain relief. We took X-rays, cleaned, and dressed her finger. I informed her mom that she needed to go to the trauma center immediately for a hand surgeon consult and further evaluation. I even faxed (ha!) and called the ER with her history to try to speed up her wait time.

When I called the next day to check on her, her father answered the phone and immediately began berating me. He asked me why we "didn't do anything for her" and sent her to the hospital. His family had come to us many times before and had no idea why we couldn't surgically repair her hand. Holding back a strong urge to say *please go fuck yourself*, instead I said, "You know what, your daughter is eighteen years old, could you put her on the phone please?"

When my patient took the phone, she was clearly groggy from pain medication and I asked her how her finger was. She informed me that it was "terrible, still bleeding, and still in pain."

"What did the hand surgeon say?"

"They didn't call one."

"Why not?"

"I don't know, they just sewed it up."

"Really, that's it?"

"Uh, no. I have an appointment with a plastic surgeon next week [sometimes plastic surgeons are trained as hand specialists] and I'm supposed to go back to the hospital today if it's not improving."

"Oh, you did get a specialist consultation and have a follow-up then?"

"I guess so . . . I was stuck there for hours and they

didn't care about your stupid phone call!"

Glad I asked. I was concerned you might lose your dominant hand's thumb. You're upset that I'm not a board-certified hand surgeon posing as a PA.

Make sure you check the thumbs-up box when we send you the survey.

Long Flight

A female in her midthirties arrived at the clinic with sudden shortness of breath and chest pain. She was taking birth control pills and had recently taken a long flight back from Europe, a classic presentation of a pulmonary embolism (or PE, a blood clot in your lungs). About 10%–30% of all PEs result in death within a month, *not a great diagnosis to miss.*[21]

After the cursory negative chest X-ray and EKG, I laid out the simple case to her and her husband for going to the ER for a CT scan of her chest, the only test that would definitively provide an answer. The primary reason: *avoidance of death.*

"No, I don't think so."

"Why is that?"

"There's no way I have a blood clot; I'm very healthy."

"Then why are you short of breath, why does your chest hurt?"

"I don't have one. I'm going to go home and rest. C'mon, honey."

At this point I made a last gasp appeal to her husband.

---

[21] "Pulmonary embolism deaths, disparities high despite advancements in care," University of Michigan Institute For Healthcare Policy & Innovation, August 31, 2023, https://ihpi.umich.edu/news-events/news/pulmonary-embolism-deaths-disparities-high-despite-advancements-care.

"You guys have kids, right?"

"Yes."

"Do you want to raise them by yourself?"

Six hours later, I called my patient. She had been admitted to the hospital with a pulmonary embolism.

"How are you feeling?"

"My chest still hurts; thanks for ruining my day."

Click.

Indigestion

A few times a week a middle-aged or elderly patient walks in, usually after dinner, looking like death. They tell me that they're having chest pain and they "want to make sure it's not a heart attack."

Why would it be? You're fifty pounds overweight, you've already had a heart attack, and it feels just like the last time you had one!

But no, tonight is different.

When I go through the motions and present them with a copy of a terribly abnormal EKG, pop some chewable aspirin into their mouths, and call 9-1-1, there is usually an argument.

"I don't want to stay in the hospital. Do I have to go?"

"Yes, the ambulance is on the way."

"Can I at least go home first to get my clothes?"

"No, you're having a **HEART ATTACK**. You have to go with the paramedics, *now*."

"This is ridiculous. It's just indigestion."

When I reach for the phone two days later, my patient informs me that he indeed had his second heart attack, and was still admitted to the cardiac unit. Was there a thank you? Was there a "Gee, you were right"?

Nah.

"I want you to know that as soon as I'm released from the hospital I'll be sending your company a letter not only requesting my money back, but asking you to pay for my hospital bill as well. I never would've been stuck here if I didn't come to your office!"

You're right.

You'd currently be financing your own funeral.

The Belly Button Callback

I feel obligated to mention this.

It's not me placing a follow-up call this time. It's an angry parent of a minor whose teenage daughter was seen last night with an infected belly button ring. Not unlike being shot or stepping on a nail, when your piercing is the source of infection, the treatment, as any layperson might guess, is to remove the foreign object.

"I laid out three hundred dollars for my twelve-year-old daughter to have her navel pierced, and dammit, I want to leave that fake rhinestone in!"

I have already explained this to the parent and patient, written them antibiotics, and recommended thorough cleaning and soaking of the wound.

"But are you sure it needs to come out? She just got it!"

"Yes, as it turns out, your belly button is not an area of your body that's meant to have two holes put through it. Her body is rejecting it."

"What if we leave it in?"

"Then you can go somewhere else when your daughter has a fever of a hundred and three, and there's so much pus and infection that you won't physically be able to remove the ring."

"What about Mudfest? Mudfest!"

I hung up the phone, defeated again.

And I assure you, *Mudfest* is a real thing.

The Timeline: Part 3

1200–1230:

Some days you think it can't get any worse, and then there's September 11th. Every second for the past three hours has been a micro universe of stress, duty, and fear. Displaced from my memory, the goodbye kiss I gave my fiancée, Lori, a few hours earlier. Before she grabbed a car service to La-Guardia to catch a plane for Pittsburgh.

Like a twisted Wachowski plot, I have to find a phone, *a real phone*. While my Nokia 5165 fails to find a signal (and I might be dead by the time I hit each button three times to send a text), I sprint up the pier in search of a pay-phone bank. Desperation leads me to race inside the doors of an abandoned cruise-line office.

One hard line still functions. *Dial Tone.*

And then more pain.

Lori's phone *beep beep beep.*

Her office hasn't heard from her or anyone on her team flying to Pittsburgh that morning. No confirmation that her plane has arrived. Empty calls to my mom and brothers.

Tick tick tick.

Shit.

One more try to Lori's phone. Straight to voicemail, an indication of nothing more than maybe a cellphone tower being restored or a temporary glitch. I pour out as much love as I have before the buzzer cuts me off. My voice evidence enough that I am still alive.

Oblivious at first to non-EMS personnel, the Piers are buzzing with NYPD, FBI, and box trucks backing into loading docks. Cots, medical supplies, food, and communications equipment stream out into what is becoming a makeshift triage area and surgical hospital. Again, *where are the wounded?* It is clear now that this is also being staged as a makeshift morgue.

When I finally return from my frantic calls, I find Steve leaning against the bus. Miraculously, he has retrieved his voicemails. He gives me an assuring look and places a strong hand on my shoulder as he gives me the news.

Lori is okay.

It wasn't her plane that crashed. His dad is alive. Lori is alive.

I haven't used any tears, and emotionally all I have left to give is anger. As adrenaline wanes, it's more than enough.

It's only 12:30.

1302–1500:

The strangest hours of the day.

Is it over?

Is it just beginning?

Ravenous to do something, I approach an FDNY boss. *Let us go, man. Let us go.* I assume that Steve and I will be running a shuttle back and forth from the towers to Chelsea Piers, and when that fills up, to whoever has a free stretcher. We haven't moved in an hour. We haven't moved in two hours. Boss clicks his radio out of indifference.

No Go.

It does not occur to me that it is a binary event. *Survive/Not Survive.* Too devastating to believe. At three o'clock, dispatch pulls us, 10 Frank, from the Piers to return to 9-1-1 calls or to simply be available. Steve and I are crushed. As we loop down the Piers exit to painfully turn north, we pass volley ambulances, displacing us from what is rightfully our fucking job.

With each block up the West Side Highway, we know that one more street and maybe one more unit stand between us and ever returning to Ground Zero today. Disgusted and defeated, we arrive back at 77th and Lex.

1600–1637:
Nobody knows what to do.

A stress debriefing with an anxious and angry bunch of terrorism survivors is stressing the fuck out of everyone.

Our crew quarters are more Sweathogs Locker Room than Lenox Hill chic. Stale BO and clinging smoke mixed with microwaved Chinese food and overcompensating cologne. While celebrities like Sarah Jessica Parker give birth in private suites across the street, we lug dirty equipment bags up the narrow steps to a converted and outdated pre-war apartment. Two overused bathrooms on the right. Straight ahead are the supervisors' "offices," where I am often called in for heckling.

As the only Midwesterner of the bunch, I never could quite get New York slang down. Instead of "my wife is fucking me (over)," I'd say, "my wife fucked me this weekend." Kenny and Manny always have a good laugh at my expense. Tony never laughs at anything.

On the left are our lockers. Most hang open (nobody steals from each other here) with dangling Yankees hats, Top Ramen cups, extra layers, even pullovers from second EMS jobs. There is an alcove with a pull-up bar and replacement parts for our gear. Vomit bins, even larger vomit bins, IV bags, needles, and ace wraps fill endless racks. And we are jammed into every inch.

We scream in relief with raised fists every time a medic comes up the steps. Will and Tom and Liz, fuck yeah! Those covered with the most ash have been closest to death. We hug the shit out of each other. But Steve and I remain attached, a singular surviving entity.

As Kenny and John thank us and hand out water bottles, *rage* washes over me.

I had almost been murdered.

By complete strangers.

My partner, my future wife, my friends. I have witnessed murder in blunt force and various forms of torture. I have seen humans falling from the sky and dead bodies on the ground. I have been ripped from my burning city, forced to watch it smolder while tauntingly in reach.

As equipped as anyone to help, feeling an invincible glow with Steve by my side. And rendered useless.

Would these guys shut the fuck up already!

The *disquiet*.

White noise about trauma and mental health resources grate on us as Steve and I inch towards the hallway.

CISD?

PTSD?

Listen, motherfuckers. Every minute of this day is an extra life for me! *I have already survived.* So to contemplate where my brain might be a day or a month from now is insanity.

Why are we fucking standing around!?!

The *helplessness*.

The survival entity Adam/Steve snaps.

People are dying as we stand here.

We know it.

American Triage

We *know* it.

We explode down the steps and back into the bus. We are our own unit now, 10 Fucking Us, dispatch. Driving recklessly and aimlessly towards Ground Zero, hoping to not get stopped. Hoping to help just one, anyone.

Please.

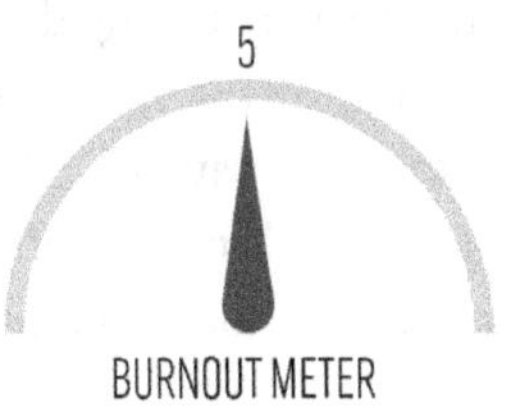

Can I Go Running Tomorrow?

South Florida 2010s

"It's my ankle, my knee, both knees actually."

"How did you hurt yourself?"

"I was jumping."

"You were working out?"

"No, I was jumping on the sidewalk. I caught the edge and rolled my ankle."

"I thought you said your knees hurt?"

"They do. I twisted my ankle and fell onto my left knee."

"What about your right knee?"

"Oh, that one hurts worse."

"Did you even injure it?"

"I think so."

"I'm not going to x-ray your whole body, and knee X-rays aren't going to tell us if you tore something. Why don't we start by x-raying your ankle?"

"I don't know, I'm in a lot of pain."

"I'm not saying [although I'd like to] that you're not in pain, I'm saying that we won't gather much information from an X-ray."

A few minutes after him shuffling down the hall for his X-ray with no trace of a limp, the rad tech popped her head out. "He wants both knees X-rayed."

Of course he does. I couldn't contain my disgust as he almost galloped back to his room, smug in his naive contentment.

"Hey, we discussed that those X-rays were a waste of time."

"I know, but I wanted to make sure I was okay."

I followed him back into the room and closed the door. "No, I didn't mean a waste of your time. I meant a waste of *our* time. You took my rad tech out of commission for an extra fifteen minutes to perform a bunch of useless tests that we had already discussed would not in any way aid our diagnosis. Nothing is broken. Let's get you a pair of crutches and have you follow-up with ortho if you're in that much pain."

"Oh, nothing's broken? So, can I go running tomorrow?"

"Running? Look man, make up your mind! Either you hurt yourself or you didn't. You told me you couldn't sleep last night because you were in too much pain, and now, after requiring full lower-body X-rays, you want to know if you can go running tomorrow?"

Speaking of pain, unfortunately, mine was not over for the evening.

"Did you tell this guy he could come back if he wasn't improving, at no charge?"

"No, I didn't tell him that."

"Are you sure?"

"Yes, I'm sure for two reasons. First, I never tell *anybody* that. And second, I remember this guy. He had a GI issue, which we discussed at length."

"He wants to know if you'll write him an antibiotic . . ."

"I know what he wants; tell him he has to pay again if he wants to be seen."

A few minutes later I'm confronted with the same guy who had made up the story about me telling him to come back for his diarrhea.

"Hey, what are you doing here? I thought you were going to see your GI doctor, like we discussed, if you weren't getting better."

"I think I'm still having the same symptoms. After I took the medicine you gave me, I didn't move my bowels for three days. Now I'm having snakelike stools."

"But the diarrhea is gone, which is why you came in a couple of days ago."

"I don't know, now I'm having some cramps and really bad gas, so, that to me, is still kinda like the diarrhea I came in for."

"No, that's completely the *opposite* of diarrhea. You said you didn't move your bowels for three days."

"Okay, maybe it's not the same thing. How's about you give me the antibiotic and we'll be all set. I'll try to see my doctor next week."

"No, you told me you would see your doctor *this* week, and here you are with a different GI complaint, but still requesting the same treatment. We don't treat nebulous abdominal pain with antibiotics 'just in case.' If you're in that much pain, you should go to the hospital."

"I'm not in too much pain, but I don't want to go the whole weekend without having medicine in case it gets worse."

"In case what gets worse? You don't have diarrhea!"

"So you're not gonna help me just because I didn't listen to you last time?"

"I did help you."

"Ya, so, where are we on that antibiotic?"

"ER. Home. Those are your two choices, that's where we are."

"I ain't going to the ER, there are sick people and diseases there. I guess I'll go home. You better hope I don't get worse."

"If you do, you know where to go . . ."

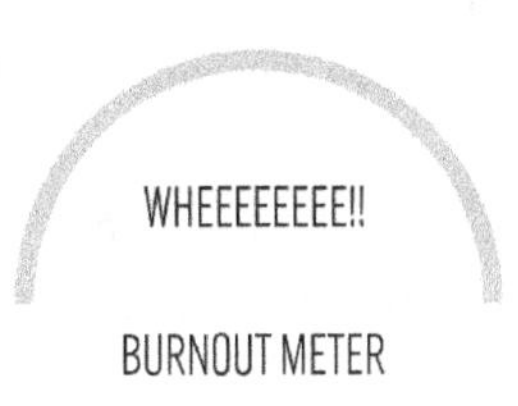

Times Square

Manhattan, 2002

Rob isn't my regular partner. Which is good, because I'm not sure I can run like this every shift. He's the biggest "buff" in the Lenox Hill crew, a medic who grabs any interesting call in our area whether he's assigned or not. You can routinely hear his deep Guyanese voice over EMS radio, making laughable excuses to magically appear only a few blocks away from the action. He took pity on me, or at least liked fucking with me, from day one. On more than one occasion, he serenaded me while I was in the crew bathroom from his ambulance mic down below on E. 77th Street:

"AAAAAAAAxxxxxLLLLLeRRRRR!"

Five calls deep into an eight-hour evening shift, we are finally parked in solitude near the East River. Cool and dark enough to shut the bus off and let the special smells of Manhattan waft through open windows. Rob lowers his baseball hat to catch a nap, but props his private PD radio on the dash. Constant chatter interrupts the Yankees game and a suddenly quiet EMS evening.

Not for long though.

"Assault, Times Square. Possible double stabbing. Units please respond."

This was PD radio, and Times Square is way out of our designated area. Six other EMS units are closer to the job. Fun night in the city though.

Without lifting his brim, Rob eases the mic from the cradle.

Kccchhhhh. "10 Young. We're on that assault in Times Square. Seven minutes out."

Dispatch responds, "Repeat, 10 Young, we don't have a . . . wait, here it is. Assault Times Square. Any units closer?"

Rob is relentless. "10 Young. Six minutes out."

Shit. Better start the ambulance.

"Rob, what the f . . ."

"CLEVELAND, DRIVE!!"

In an almost-blackout type of trance, I drive our boxy beast from the river towards the bright lights in Midtown. The wrong direction down one-way streets, over sidewalks, in an effort to keep up with Rob's progressive lies to dispatch about our location.

"10 Young, ETA 3 minutes."

"We're still on the East Side, Rob!"

"Better drive faster then, Cleveland!"

Challenge accepted.

As Rob picks up the mic and berates pedestrians and cabbies for having the nerve to block our path, I navigate across town like a Frogger champion. Emerging from the bowels of the West 40s into Times Square, I skid the bus to a stop inside the crime scene.

What I remember most isn't the bleeding knife wound. Our patient winces in pain, but he's in decent shape. A fairly deep inch-wide gouge into his left lower abdomen. Vital organs intact and moderate bleeding controlled well with firm pressure dressings. The other bus has their patient in stable condition (can't exactly put the guys who stabbed each other in the same ambulance).

With a dozen officers and hundreds of curious tourists watching, we go through the backbreaking process of loading the patient and stretcher into the bus. Catch the stretcher on a notch in the ambulance floor while one medic lifts and the other pushes the wheels up to fold the legs. Finally, a giant heave forward, hoping you clear the gate without cracking anyone's head open. Barbaric (and outdated; now they're hydraulic!).

Doors open to the world, Rob uses his shears to cut through bloodied T-shirt and pants, searching for hidden knife wounds. As I hop down, I take a second to absorb the surreal. Before leaving Cleveland, I only had a few dozen suburban EMS calls under my belt. Now, I am working a double stabbing under a *Lion King* billboard you can see from outer space, barely two years later.

"10 Young, en route to Roosevelt."

I clear the chaos and turn the bus towards the hospital. With Times Square finally behind us, Rob scares the shit out of me by sliding the small window open between the front and patient compartments.

"AXLER!!!"

"What?! Is everything ok?"

Hideously deep laughter precedes Rob's complete disregard for the poor stabbed guy with two IVs hanging from his arms.

"Seven minutes! You got us there in seven fucking minutes, Ax . . ." He can't finish, he's laughing too hard.

Finally back at the Lenox Hill crew room, other medics want the gory details. How much blood? Did you see the knife? And what the hell were you doing in Times Square?

Oh, you're working with *Rob*.

I start my tale by telling everyone what an asshole he is, but I'm cut off.

"I never thought we'd stay on the call! Cleveland, driving over sidewalks! Seven minutes . . ." His wheezing laughter trails the room with him as he grabs IVs to restock the bus.

"Your first stabbing, Axler," Sylvia teases, "you'll always remember it."

No, I'll remember the *fucking ride*.

Meat

Port St. Lucie ER, Florida 2005

No, you're not a number. You're meat. That's right. Corned beef, pastrami on rye, ham and Swiss. That's how the makers of medicine and the hospital administrators of the world view you. Driving home after a twelve-hour PA school shift, I received an unexpected phone call. It was from a recruiter who represented the ownership of the company that ran the emergency room.

The ER is often the most profitable part of the hospital, sometimes owned by private companies that provide the docs, PAs, and billing. He told me the doctors and the medical director were impressed with my work and that they were considering offering me a job. But he had one important question to ask.

"Adam, can you move the meat?"

In subsequent interviews, they would repeat this mantra to me.

Can you move the meat?

Can you see forty patients in a day?

Can you sew up five patients while managing five

more?

Can you step right out of school and continue to do it day or night?

When I interviewed for my first urgent care job, the owner said the same thing.

"I don't care that you have no experience, I don't care what you've done in the past. Can you move the meat?"

At the end of my first shift at that urgent care, the doc I was working with turned to me and said, "Hey dude, nice job. You can really move the meat!"

I knew that my days in the ER were probably numbered when I got into a fight with both the charge nurse and the ER manager at the same time. I asked her how I could possibly have a ninety-eight-year-old woman with a fucking neck fracture, three abdominal pains, and a potential heart attack sitting in the express care area of the emergency room.

"I'm sitting on at least two admissions, possibly five. Anyone up there having a stroke maybe? Why don't you send them to Fast Track too!"

"Go see patients, Adam. We're busy."

"You're the one who triaged the ninety-eight-year-old from EMS right? How the hell did she get past you?"

"I'm grabbing the ER manager."

"Good. Ask him if he knows what 'dumping' means!"

The sloth-like creature, who hid most of the day in his office on the opposite corner of the ER, slowly made his way over. I made a point to bump into him.

"What's the problem, Adam?" he snarled.

"I can read the tracker. There's only twelve patients in the main ER and three docs. I'm full and have three more in the waiting room. Broken neck. Did she mention the broken neck?"

　　　　　　　　　　　　American Triage

"See patients, Adam. That's what we hired you for."

"I'm doing *my* job. What the fuck are you doing?"

The rage boiled over his half-bald head, and he almost, almost put a finger into my chest. Trying to show off for the nurse, then thought better of it. I headed back to Fast Track for my ass-kicking; he headed back to his sandwich.

They didn't want to hear that I was concerned about my patients; they wanted me to sit down, shut up, and guess what?

Move the meat.

The Google Geniuses

"Sir, we changed out the timing belt and a few of the plugs. Everything seems to be working fine now; that noise is gone."

"Really? I thought it was going to be the struts and maybe a battery terminal connection!"

What I know about fixing cars could fit into a thimble, and yet this scenario happens to me in medicine every day. It would be like me challenging my mechanics who own a Japanese racing car team about what's causing the problem (they tell me they go through the same shit too). It would be like me questioning the manner in which a three-star chef makes his crème brûlée by asking the waiter to go back in the kitchen to tell him to use more vanilla next time.

The proliferation of information through sites like WebMD (now through AI-enhanced searches), the availability of technical programs through community colleges, institutes, and even web-based universities, have given the false sense to people that they have insight into medicine.

They don't.

When someone who has "done their own research" tries to tell me what their diagnosis and treatment plan should be, it drives me insane. Even worse is when they try to use that little bit of knowledge in an effort to trap you into an incorrect diagnosis, such as this scenario.

The interview began innocently enough. A teenager had a small rash on her arm, and I asked both her and her mother a few routine questions.

When did the rash start?

Has the patient traveled recently?

Any recent antibiotic use or new medications?

Does she remember being bitten by anything?

Was she playing outside?

All of which she answered, *No.*

Her mom, apparently annoyed that I was doing my job, said, "Let me show you what the rash looked like earlier in the day."

"If you have a picture, I'd love to see it." She pulled out her iPhone and showed me a picture from the rash twelve hours ago. The rash looked almost the same with maybe a little bit of central clearing (no redness) at that time.

"I'm not exactly sure what it is, but it looks like a pretty routine rash that we can treat with a cream a couple of times a day for the next few weeks."

I could tell from the look on her face that this was not going to be an acceptable treatment and by the time I finished, I could see that she was dying to speak.

"You don't think it's a target lesion, do you?"

"*A target lesion*, like from a deer tick bite?" I asked.

"Yes, a target lesion or a bullseye lesion." Oh, she was laying on her impressive medical knowledge now and, wait for it, "because I showed it to an ER doc and he thought it was a target lesion."

Haha, you've trapped me now!

You came in under the guise of seeking routine medical treatment for your daughter, but you've had an agenda to prove me wrong from the onset. You were going to tell me what the diagnosis is, having already consulted someone else.

"You've already been to the ER today? If that's what the doctor thought then you should follow their advice."

"*She* wasn't in the ER, but I did show the picture to an ER doctor after looking it up on Google [the same university McCarthy went to!]. I work at the hospital, you know [I do know, because you've mentioned it three times]."

"Why isn't the doctor providing treatment for you then? Did he offer to write her a prescription?"

"No, like I said, he didn't see her but he thought that she should be treated for it."

This whole visit has been a farce. She's not interested in my medical opinion because she has already determined that this is Lyme disease.

"You're here for antibiotics to treat Lyme disease; that's really why you came."

"Don't *you* think it's a target lesion?"

"We don't live in a state that has deer ticks [the carriers for Lyme], so there are no local cases. You told me that you haven't traveled to any endemic areas, and there has been no tick attached to your daughter's arm at any point or even a bite that we know of. If you want my opinion, no, I don't think it's the beginning of Lyme disease."

"The ER doctor is wrong then? *Google* is wrong?"

"No, I didn't say he was wrong. I'm saying he didn't even examine your daughter and this here does not look like a target lesion. But I can see that you're here for a di-

agnosis of Lyme disease and that you're going to be upset
if I don't offer you treatment.

"Why don't we do this?

"Let me write you the cream, which I think will help
your daughter, and also write you the prophylaxis for Lyme
disease. We're not going to do any testing for it here; we'll
leave that up to your pediatrician. You can follow up with
them in a couple of days."

"I don't understand. Are you writing me the medication because you think that's what I want or because you
think that my daughter might have Lyme disease?"

"Now I'm confused. I thought we discussed that I didn't
think that she has Lyme disease but you expressed concern
that my opinion was wrong because you have already consulted someone *or something* else. I'm actually offering you
the treatment that you're here for."

Things only got worse after that. A few minutes later,
the pharmacy called asking to change the dosage on the
prescription because they didn't have it in stock. After
consulting the doctor, we agreed to change the dosage to
something else that was still in the correct range with the
full knowledge of mom, who was standing right next to the
pharmacist.

The next day there was a call to complain, of course,
that my diagnosis had been incorrect, that she needed the
doctor to review the chart, and that I had written a "subtherapeutic" dosage of the medication, which according to
all the literature was simply not true.

But as is apt to happen in the customer-service world
of medication, we rewrote the dosage I had originally written the night before that the pharmacist couldn't fill with
the mother's full knowledge, and called that in again. We
were now back to the third dosage of the medication that

this patient didn't need in the first place.

The following day, a call would come in to complain that the dosage of the medication for the disease that her daughter didn't have was too expensive and that she would like to revert back to the subtherapeutic dosage that she had called to complain about the previous day. Apparently, it was therapeutic now that it was in the right price range. Boom, presto, our fourth change of the same medication, back to the dose that she didn't want the day before.

Did we remind her of this?

Of course not, the minions took the order and filled it while our manager hung her head in shame.

The "art of medicine"?

Haha, laugh along with me.

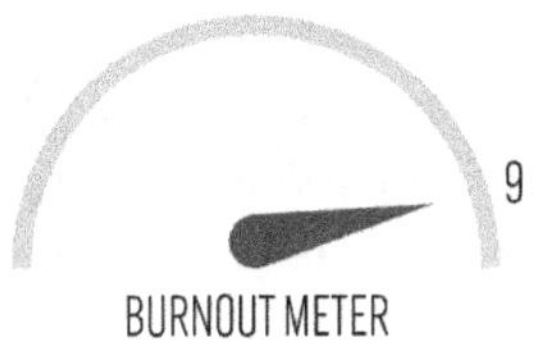

Tips for Drug Seekers

Anywhere U.S.A. 2019

The most comprehensive list ever assembled for scoring legal controlled substances from your doctor and not having them throw you in jail in the process:

1. Have a real injury that includes either uncontrolled bleeding or a bone sticking through your skin.
2. Do not show up with your MRI films.
3. Do not show up with your mommy.
4. Do not show up with your small children in an effort to gain sympathy. This will only make you appear to be a degenerate.
5. Do not show up with your drug-seeking spouse/girlfriend who does all the talking for you with her clearly constricted/dilated pupils.
6. Do not show up with sunglasses at eight o'clock at night.
7. Do not ask for a wheelchair because you're in too much pain.
8. Dental pain is a dental problem, not a medical

problem. You can even ask Medicare about this one.

9. Rating your pain as a 20 out of 10 will get you sent to the emergency room, not narcotics.

10. Cover your track marks by wearing long sleeves or a jacket.

11. Don't be from out of town.

12. Don't tell me that your purse/wallet/backpack/luggage was stolen.

13. Don't be between the ages of eighteen and fifty-nine.

14. Don't tell me you were "jumped," as evidenced by your black-and-blue marks, but can't remember when and where, and that you didn't call the police. I'll be happy to do it for you.

15. Don't be allergic to tramadol.

16. Don't be allergic to Tylenol as a component of your pain medicine because we know immediately this means you intend to snort it or shoot it.

17. Don't tweak in front of me.

18. Don't tell me that your doctor is dead, your pet is dead, your mother is dead, that your wife is dead, or that anyone you know has died recently.

19. Don't stutter when I ask you if you've ever taken medicine that has worked for you before like P-P-Percocet.

20. Don't ask me for medicine to help you sleep. I always have the same answer for that, Benadryl.

21. Don't threaten to not pay if I don't write you narcotics.

22. Don't tell me that you "work in medicine" and are requesting controlled substances.

23. Don't show up with your drug addict friends and

giggle in the waiting room before we call you.

24. Don't tell me that you ran out of your pain meds and that your doctor is out of town.
25. Don't act like it's common to take methadone or Roxicodone.
26. Don't have eight addresses in the narcotics database.
27. Don't say, "It's not touching it."
28. Don't forget the last time when I told you I wouldn't write you narcotics.
29. If your doctor "always" writes you dope, then why don't you call them?

If I'm forgetting anything, I'm sure there's a holiday weekend coming up that will remind me.

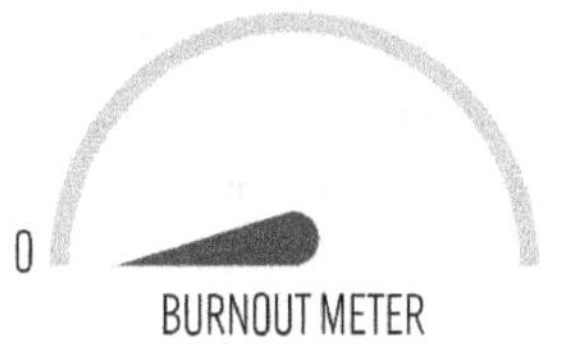

Cleveland FNG

Mentor, Ohio 1998

"Get in the fucking truck, Axler."

A month before the September 11th attacks, my best friend, Rock, made the nearly ten-hour drive from Cleveland for our annual New York locals tour of dive bars, pizza, and a chance to add some curios to his collection. I couldn't get my Sunday shift at Lenox Hill switched, so Lori took Rock downtown. He borrowed my subway MetroCard and they spent that August 2001 afternoon hanging in Chinatown and SoHo before heading for one last stop. A Demon Drop elevator ride up to the 107th floor of the North Tower for a view from Windows on the World.

Four weeks before the restaurant and tower would no longer exist.

Four weeks before I would become one of the very few medics to work and survive 9/11.

Only a few years earlier, I was getting my ass handed to me in Cleveland at the Mentor Fire Department as the FNG (fucking new guy) . . .

The only thing louder than fire alarm bells raging inside Station 5, was the sucking sound emanating from a late '80s model Hoover. Diligently being pushed into the corners of the chief's office before I mopped the floors and replaced the trash. Along with shaving twice a day to appease encrusted former-military-turned-FD lieutenants, this was not exactly the excitement I signed up for. *It blew.*

As I returned the vacuum to the closet, I noticed only the lieutenant and the ladder company remained in the kitchen. The ambulance and engine were mysteriously missing from their bays.

Painfully, all I could gulp out was, "I missed the bells, huh?"

Thankfully, Lt. Roberts never took me that seriously so he chuckled, muttered something about "FNGs," and he made a mental note. Still happy to be employed, I made sure to not even think about taking a piss the rest of the week for fear of missing a call. I spent my lunch hours practicing putting on my gear and rolling hose. Certainly not my last fuckup in my first job in EMS.

Wrapping up a routine house call a week later, I put the O2 bag back into the ambulance. But before I could settle into the passenger seat, I felt a vice grip on my forearm and looked back.

Lt. Roberts said, "You're driving."

"The Engine?"

I had barely graduated to driving the ambulance, so when I was asked to take the wheel of a real fire truck, something you need actual training for, I protested in the name of public safety (mainly my own). This was OJT for the FNG, an unscheduled probation test that brought a smile to the lieutenant's face.

American Triage

I reluctantly climbed into the driver's seat, strapped into what was only a lap belt, and tried to figure out how to move something with a horizontal wheel for the first time in my life. The seat was a bony metal, barely covered in leather scraps. Like Toonces gathering his bearings, I could barely reach the pedals, and truthfully would've been more comfortable driving this thing standing up.

After stalling as long as I could, I looked over to the lieutenant and gave a shrug that could only be translated as *"what the fuck?"*

A panel of green switches, push/pull buttons, and a traditional key ignition apparently had to be manipulated in some sort of magical order to crank this thing up. Lou reached over, popped a switch, slammed a button down and told me to turn the key.

The control panel flared with enthusiastic dings.

The brakes hissed a sigh of relief and the distinctly diesel beast roared to life.

My ass started vibrating.

And for a moment I thought, this is fucking cool!

Oh shit, I still have to drive.

I gingerly pushed down on the skinny pedal and the engine laughed at me, not moving an inch. I applied more pressure and still no action.

Fuck it.

I stood up with all my weight and lurched us forward, before slamming the brake in panic. Like teaching one of my teen daughters how to drive, the engine mushed forward in a series of half lunges and sudden stops. While Roberts went pale with regret, I was getting the hang of it and I eased us onto a local road.

What he didn't tell me as I headed for a red light and my first encounter with a car, was how to brake properly.

I jammed my foot down but we kept moving, closer and closer to an unsuspecting minivan. It turns out Newton was right. Five hundred gallons of water slammed up against the cabin and jolted me forward into the antiquated wheel. Half-standing, the brakes were on the floor and we pulled up inches from a crash.

This wasn't a joyride in a new toy. Angled turns through cul-de-sacs, cutting through the Giant Eagle parking lot, and getting up to speed through traffic on Center Street. White knuckled and hunched over the wheel, hoping for instructions to head back to headquarters while surviving my biggest probie challenge yet.

In NYC, I once took the mirrors off eight triple-parked cars in a row, squeezing down an East 80s street to get to our patient. But this was a suburban fire department and a quarter-million-dollars worth of equipment. I felt like I was playing chicken with the endless rows of mailboxes while trying not to shit my pants.

Somehow, I navigated that beast back to Station 5, cracking 50 mph once or twice and avoiding catastrophe. I always thought it was cool to see the engine pull around and through the rear bay doors, ready to face forward for the next call. Nobody was more surprised than the bat chief to see *me* behind the wheel this time.

I pulled the hydraulic brake, turned off the ignition, and flipped the master switch down. Soaked in sweat and seemingly unsoiled, I jumped down to the bay floor. Letting Lt. Roberts lead the way, I searched out and high-fived the fuck out of everyone.

On a recent trip home back to Cleveland, Rock surprised me with a sacred score from one of our all-day subway hopping and ill-fated Bloody Mary drinking contests on the Lower East Side. If we didn't make a stop at Junior's first, it was Ray's Original or H&H. But before Rock would go on to set a record for puking in three boroughs in less than thirty minutes, we always made a stop at the now defunct Ricky's.

Ricky's was like the Spencer Gifts of New York City. Aisles and aisles of pure tourist-trap crap, enticing the naive to drop Midwestern dollars here instead of a street hustler's stand. Rock always refused to leave the city before purchasing a bauble for his collection.

As I reached into the brown paper bag, I could only hope to find the best NYC nostalgia ever created. Still stamped with the original $5.99 price tag, it was *The Devil's Magic 8 Ball*. Purchased because even in the package you could shake it and be rewarded with advice from the dark lord. His best words of wisdom?

DO IT YOU COWARD!

I laughed hard enough to cry as I cracked open the package, committing collectibles suicide and earning a groan. I shook the devil furiously, but its mystery fluid had long dried up and the words had become a hazy paste. I didn't give a fuck, I was too happy that almost twenty-five years later Lori and Rock were alive.

And I sure as hell was no coward on *that* day.

The Timeline: Part 4

1700:

It's five o'clock.

Dispatch caught between terrorist attack and heart attack.

Four hundred jobs are holding in Manhattan, most people either having the common decency to not call 9-1-1 with minor bullshit or too terrified to leave their own apartments. A million people suddenly in need of a Xanax (truly in need); so many palpitations and nervous breakdowns.

Steve and I pick up a cardiac call, thrilled to transport a patient to the covered bay at Cornell. As we pull in, a line of stretchers staged outside the ER doors. Expectant doctors and nurses each with the hopeful look of a child waiting for a parent in an after-school pick-up line. And the same disappointing look as a car passes them by when we wheel our "regular" patient through the doors.

The same scene plays out on our next few calls, working a scattered four jobs in the next eight hours.

Empty beds.

Empty ERs.

And thinking about how lonely the unusually placed stretchers outside our Lenox Hill doors are as we come and go. I know now that a binary event has occurred.

Anyone who could make it, made it.

Anyone who couldn't, is *dead*.

0118:

I don't want to get out of the car. Steve gives me a ride home, a few blocks away and unnecessary, but we know that when we say goodnight, the survival entity Adam/Steve dies with this day. I have an empty apartment waiting, and he faces a ghastly drive back to Long Island. "Get home safe," seems vacuous, so I pull out the keys to my walkup and say "Thank you."

0130–0200:

The answering machine beeps in anger. I ignore it, not ready for more pain. After showering off bits of tower and blood, I finally find the balls to hit play.

I listen to Mom and Dad. I listen to Rock. I listen to Lori's friends and parents. I listen to Craig from the Mentor FD. I listen to my brothers. When I feel I can put a sentence together, I call my older brother, Noah, at 2 a.m. to relive the day.

The tears don't flow . . . more like *flood out*, in one big Harvey Keitel grunting wail.

0600–0800:

I clutch the phone and briefly sleep, only because exhaustion forces me to. The news plays on loop in the background. Each time the towers start burning, I picture myself on a surreal map with the caption: **YOU ARE HERE**.

Wednesday, my off day. I brush my teeth and put on clean BDUs, a T-shirt, and my Lenox Hill baseball hat. Getting in and out of the city is a physical impossibility,

                    American Triage

but I can walk to work, and that's what I do.
I am no longer in NYC.
I am at the center of the fucking world.
It's September 12th, eight o'clock.

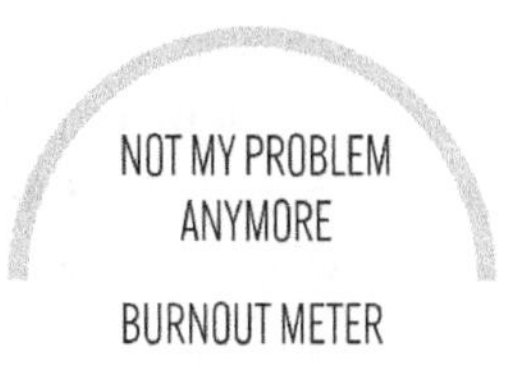

From 9/11 to *Fahrenheit 451*

Sarasota, Florida

Vulcan's Hammer and *Dr. Futurity.* The titles alone were nerd-bait enough. But Emsh's Paul Newmanesque and Valigursky's hand-painted spaceships on Philip K. Dick's Ace Double covers called to me through A. Parker's Books' spotlight case. The colorful wraps were true works of art, nudged by PKD's once-in-a-universe genius, only subtly hinting at the treasures inside. I greedily grabbed both 1960 first-edition paperbacks for the journey home.

Lori's and my first vacation alone without our two young daughters to Sarasota and St. Armands was memorable for two things.

First, upon returning home we discovered a large sign posted above our alarm box inside the front door. It was our "secret" code, boldly written in large numbers by my in-laws. Certainly helpful to them, as well as any would-be intruders. I could only hope that those same intruders would also help them with making instant oatmeal. As that was one of several consulting calls that vibrated our vacationing phones. And thus ended any hope of traveling without our girls for the next decade.

The second, however, was the reinvigoration of my love of reading and collecting incredible books, particularly editions with great covers. Sure, I always had a beat-up copy of Dick's *High Castle*, Tim Powers's *Last Call*, *Lord of the Rings* box sets, and copies of Le Guin's *Earthsea* lying around. Sherlock Holmes nesting in the nook above the TV. But chasing scientific degrees and keeping current with medical journals sapped time and creative curiosity.

The trip, though, made me realize I had starved half my mind.

The half I liked.

And I was angry about it.

My clinic days were filled with executing in the complete opposite fashion of these stories I loved so much. Hundreds of decisions. Allergies, compliance, history gathering. Was triage even done correctly? A temperature of 90.2°F on a patient (hypothermia starts around 95°F)! I asked my nurse, "Is the patient dead?" All in an effort to be *precise*. To narrow my diagnosis down a single path.

This isn't the case with the science/fantasy that grew out of pulps and prurient shadows. The Thing, The Doom, The Shadow. A single idea was all that mattered. One that could give a fuck about grammar or that had more dangling plot holes than participles.

Creativity and imagination, not cold processing.

You remember Arnold Schwarzenegger and a sweaty Sharon Stone (okay, maybe I remember that) from *Total Recall*? Only twenty pages of PKD's "We Can Remember It for You Wholesale" inspired this Martian spy adventure. Lost somewhere in the script was the best part of the story. Our hero had been gifted a magic invisible destroying rod by mouselike alien visitors. *A magic invisible destroy-*

ing rod! Something childish and fantastical, silly, and yet, you can't help but reread the story over and over, wanting nothing more than to see Douglas Quail win in the end.

Ray Bradbury's influence spans over seventy-five years now (all the way to my own subtitle). It would be impossible to read his *Something Wicked This Way Comes* and not feel the way Stephen King writes children. But it was his take on the butterfly effect that grabbed me long before *Fahrenheit 451*. "A Sound of Thunder" may even be the origin of the butterfly effect, a dinosaur time-travel story with inevitable disaster created by a single misstep.

I love the other end of the sci-fi spectrum too. Polymaths like Lem, Clarke and more recently, Cixin. Works so far ahead of their time, they almost seem like falsified documents in retrospect. Lem predicted a possible internet long before Gibson's cyberpunk masterpiece *Neuromancer*. Noted sci-fi author Kim Stanley Robinson anointed Lem's *Solaris* as being so quintessentially *the* alien story that other alien stories were no longer necessary (love you KSR, but I'm going to keep reading!). Clarke's imagined satellites and spaceships became NASA reality. And the barely comprehensible (even to mortal scientists) *Three-Body Problem* demands rereading. If nothing else, to bathe your brain in the impossible.

You could argue that Ursula K. Le Guin is not our greatest American writer, and I would laugh. Inventor of languages, multiple universes, and a boy wizard who is whisked off to magic school and haunted by a dark spirit, *thirty years* before that other kid. Writer of hard sci-fi (*The Dispossessed*), Dickian sci-fi (*The Lathe of Heaven*), and a prescient mix of feminism, sexuality, xenophobia and pure darkness (*The Left Hand of Darkness*) that still chills me.

Poetry, children's books, and essays that define genres,

all separate her writing from the mere literature that preceded her.

But it's not all aliens and electric sheep that drew me to sci-fi. Staring back from my frequently dusted shelves is Burgess's iconic one-eyed droog. There is an American teen enjoying a Coke under the shadow of the Rocky Mountains and a swastika. Pelham's lockstep imagination of Ballard's postwar England either burning or drowning, but always dying. Not in stark grays or shaded black, but in vivid color.

Memories of entire earth wars, whose victors still carried plenty of the burning embers of evil in shallow pockets. Reminders from Huxley and Orwell are all too relevant almost 100 years later. As haunting as Indiana Jones's Lost Ark being crated into a vacuous American warehouse, maybe to be lost forever.

Whether arks or crosses, another draw for me has always been the *science* in science fiction, specifically at the expense of religion. Or any belief system outside of deductive reasoning. Not only Asimov and Clarke, but James Blish's Jesuit in *A Case of Conscience*, or Harry Harrison's missionary in "The Streets of Ashkelon." Efforts to force a belief system on more intelligent beings who have already trivialized any notion of untruth or immorality. I can hear Max Von Sydow's King Osric ringing in my head, *"What outrageousness! What arrogance!"*[22]

As if a priest in any cloth could hold more truth for me than Sagan or Tiptree Jr.

Not even Bradbury could have predicted the course firefighters would take. His early '50s book burners were born out of the blatant anti-intellectualism of World War

---

[22] *Conan the Barbarian*, directed by John Milius (Universal Pictures, 1982), DVD.

  American Triage

II fascists. But in reality, it has been science and medicine that have actually kept the business of fire departments going. My first job in medicine was as a suburban firefighter/medic in Mentor, Ohio. The entire city had been brought up to fire code in the '60s and no building was more than three stories tall. New construction was more concrete than wood. Even our work pants were fire retardant and the "hoods," which once would've had you ridiculed as a firefighter, would get you fired if you didn't don them at the first hint of smoke or flame.

So what did the fire department do when there were no more fires?

They took over EMS. First, CPR and the Ghostbusters' hearse. Then, a real ambulance loaded with AEDs, IVs, and everything from Ativan to epinephrine. There are fucking cameras on the intubation kits now! Where the hell was that when I was pushing tubes through vocal cords? The priority for the department was me going to paramedic school, not fire training. While nothing was cooler than saying I was a firefighter, the job was 99% EMS.

In order to become a medic in NYC, I memorized a thick blue binder full of hundreds of protocols. Only after waiting for a passing written score did they usher you into a large conference room. There, emergency medicine MDs from the five boroughs waited to administer three oral scenarios to see if you were fit to be a NYC paramedic. Oral boards to have the privilege of working for the fire department! Almost unimaginable to the NYC of James Baldwin and Frank Sinatra.

But given enough time, Bradbury's firefighters and the brave new world have returned. The emails I get from the Florida Surgeon General read like QAnon promotional material. Perfectly happy to let retirees like my dad with

COPD and other health problems die or be forgotten by our medical system. Who needs Crichton to invent new viruses when we can bring back the old ones! Our new director of HHS is more than happy to have a measles revival.

What's next, *polio?*

And let's not forget Atwood's Handmaids. The tale of abortion law and women's bodily autonomy is reaching into medical residency. Who the fuck wants to be trained at a hospital where part of your training is *illegal?* Or establish a practice in that state? Why train at Vanderbilt or Baylor when you can opt for Berkeley or Chicago?

Fortunately, I can hit the delete button these days.

My licenses remain intact just in case, but I've been able to give more solid medical advice to my book buyers who trust me as an expert than I was able to on a daily basis in an actual clinic! Keeping up with the pseudoscientific whims of our current dystopia concerns me less than introducing my friends and customers to the fantastic and terrifying worlds between the pages of Penguin paperbacks or those Ace Doubles.

And thankfully, letting them do the same for me.

Getting out of medicine was *not* easy. Leaving a few million dollars in guaranteed earnings on the table along with lingering loans is a tough sell. Especially for this guy, who had never sold anything but beer and chicken wings.

It happened this way.

I take my scrubs off in the garage, put them right in the wash. Lt. Elmore taught me early on, never bring your work clothes home. I don't hug my daughters or Lori, not even a quick hello. I feel *dirty*, mentally and physically. At first I need ten minutes, then twenty, then, however long it takes. Before I feel clean from my shift and can be *normal* again.

Sitting quietly at dinner after I tuck the girls in, Lori says:

"Every day I expect you to come home and tell me you quit."

I look up at her, knowing I have imagined an *Office Space* scenario in my head for months. Something has to change.

I started selling my duplicate paperbacks online to support my Sci-Fi and PKD collections. Then I started contributing to The ISFDB (The Internet Speculative Fiction Database, true nerd shit). Crediting artists and sharing forgotten editions with the world.

I made an Instagram page to post my favorite covers and authors. People liked them. Ooohh, who's the artist? Where did you get that? *How much?*

And suddenly, I had followers, then customers, then, maybe a bookstore? I expanded from classic Sci-Fi and Fantasy into entirely collectible offshoots. *Heavy Metal* magazine and oversized pulps from the '30s, full of the original fantasy art masters. I grabbed Frank Frazetta covers for my crazy for Conan readers, even *Dungeons & Dragons* was back!

Then one afternoon, I drove to Vero Beach to look at a promising collection. The easygoing retiree called Samuel Delany "Chip," and knew all the lingo. As I filled box after box with saleable treasures, I found an early copy of *A Clockwork Orange.*

"Oh that one's signed. You can have it."

Signed?

As the story went, Burgess signed a bunch of copies at SUNY Orange, the retiree's alma mater, back in the early '70s. I gladly grabbed it with the rest of my haul, and as I drove home thought, who the fuck would make something like that up?

But I had to be sure. I tracked down the Cultural Affairs Coordinator at SUNY O. She said, *"Let me ask my librarian friend."* Who happened to be the wife of the retired professor who picked up Burgess from NYC and brought him to campus.

Holy Shit. I can do this.

One more thing. Lori needed a full-time job. She had worked on everything from Tums to Olympic campaigns at her NYC ad agency. But Florida was a different beast. After a year of consulting for a national real-estate developer, her boss said we need an in-house marketing department. Instead of following his search parameters, she persuaded him to "acquire" her business, Brand You. And boom, she was the Head of Marketing.

I got the call at 2:30.

"QUIT YOUR JOB."

By 2:37, I was on hold with the UnitedHealthcare HR department. By 2:39, I was now a per-diem employee, *effective immediately.*

Not one "are you sure?" Not one "have you spoken with your manager?" And certainly not one fucking "thank you."

Damn, it does feel good to be a gangsta!

Shortly after, I knew I had made it as a bookseller. Customers tell me I'm their "second favorite dealer." A librarian messaged me that following my Instagram page "is like walking into a new bookstore every day." Some of your favorite writers, musicians, artists, and actors buy books from me. I've introduced thousands of readers to Lem and Le Guin. PKD, OEB, and JGB. British artists like Pelham and Miller. The instantly recognizable beauty of a Leo and Diane Dillon cover. And tried to save authors like

Blish and Bester from being lost in time.

The common bond at the clinic was our mistreatment by patients. The fight to not work thirteen hours and get paid for twelve. And the medical system in which we were easily replaceable parts. My bond with readers is *infinite*. Any book, any author. I'm not a critic, I'm a lover. From *The Long Goodbye* to *The Lottery*, from *Frankenstein* to *Discworld*.

And those bonds extend well beyond books or collecting cool covers. I'm connected to an entire world of parents my age, with kids my age. Working through COVID with teens, managing aging parents and college admissions. *Finding a goddamn ten minutes to read![23]* The connections made through books are as intense and as satisfying as any life-saving thank you letter or homemade cake I ever received.

And without which, *American Triage* would never be possible.

---

[23] Pro tip: always have a collection of short stories in the car or your bag; no excuses!

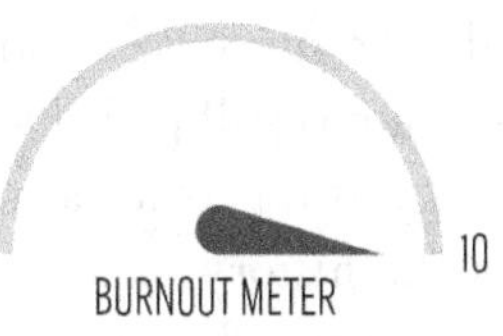

Into the Fire

This past September 11th, I held my sixteen-year-old daughter, Syd, in the inevitable Florida rain at our local memorial. A melted and twisted Tower girder rising among modern survivor plaques. Lori and I held hands and shook a little, remembering that day and what might not have been. Meanwhile, a thousand miles away, 9/11 truthers visited the actual NYC Memorial . . .

In what I can only now think parallels the changes I've seen in medicine over that time, comedian Jon Stewart stood up to become one of the staunchest supporters of rights and benefits for 9/11 survivors. And the beloved mayor Rudy Giuliani, who thanked fire and police and Port Authority but rarely EMS, lives as an outcast relic giving away his NYC apartment contents to Georgia election workers. Surreal.

More than twenty years later, I am alive and well.

I can still see black dots against the sky and am unable to turn off the switch that reminds me that those were falling victims. I can still feel the cloud from the second collapsing tower enveloping me as I ran in what felt like rubble and quicksand. The suspense of not knowing whether you had just died or not is still palpable.

But I am as lucky as it gets for a survivor of the worst terrorist attack in the history of our country. No PTSD, no asthma, no health-related issues. My daughters argue over who gets to wear my Lenox Hill and St. Luke's EMS pullovers with embroidered Axler #9749 above the hospital crests. A proud display of my badge number and a reminder that I had the privilege to work with New York City medics whose numbers were in the single and teen digits. A reminder of how lucky I am, as a member of the World Trade Center Health Registry, to have emerged mostly unscathed.

According to the registry, after two decades of research and five waves of surveys, thankfully "the majority of people exposed to the WTC attack are healthy and symptom free." However, not everyone has been as lucky as me. PTSD, asthma, depression, and decreased lung function continue to afflict WTC survivors at rates much higher than the general population. Twenty percent of people who saw the things I saw had PTSD within the first six years after 9/11. Asthma was at three times the normal rate after six years, and depression afflicted 15% of survivors ten years later.[24]

For weeks after the attacks, applause greeted our ambulance simply for showing up. Store owners came out to thank us and offer us free coffees or cold drinks. And while people shortly went back to giving us the finger, refusing to move over a lane, or complaining about sirens being too loud, it took the NYC Health Department less than two

---

[24] "What We Know - 9/11 Health," n.d., https://www.nyc.gov/site/911health/researchers/what-we-know.page.

months to create the World Trade Center Health Registry. It took less than a year to start receiving federal funding.

But as the city rebuilt, the term "hero" had been spent, and people were more annoyed about taking their shoes off at the airport than remembering tragedy, too much was forgotten. It took a *Daily Show* rampage from Stewart along with a parade of suffering survivors to move the James Zadroga 9/11 Health and Compensation Act out of filibuster purgatory and into law in 2011. Less than nine years after President Obama's signing, the house attempted to cut funding for victims by 70%. Thankfully, Stewart never lost his rage, and after he testified before the House Judiciary Committee in June of 2019 funding was restored permanently through 2090 (although the World Trade Center Health Program is underfunded and was one of the first departments cut by DOGE and HHS in 2025).

Lori and I had the privilege of volunteer bartending at a commemorative event on Roosevelt Island for those we lost, shortly after 9/11. Chosen because of my expertise serving long lines at Buffalo Wild Wings during Ohio State games and packed Cleveland nights. We took the tram across the East River and prepared for a mob like I had never seen before.

But this was no drunken post-victory celebration. This was the friendliest and slowest line of patrons to ever greet a drink. An understanding that our EMS community would never be the same, and for one night it was a wake and shivah and homegoing all at once. FDNY and medics from the Bronx to Staten shook our hands and tipped like they were putting our kids through college, knowing full well that all of the proceeds would be donated to grieving families.

Between furiously cracking open bottles of Budweiser and Bawls Soda along with some heavy pours, we drank away what was one of the happiest and saddest nights of our lives. Nobody thinking about the chronic coughs or nightmares to come. Only that I had made the right decision to go into medicine.

On a recent visit back home in Cleveland, my best friend Rock accompanied me on a bookstore and coffee tour. He reminded me of the horror in the hours and days following the September 11th attacks. Not only for me, *but for him*, and anyone who knew me. He had left one of the thirty or forty messages on my answering machine, which I wouldn't hear until staggering into my empty apartment at 1:30 a.m. early Wednesday morning.

Empty.

Without Lori.

Rock reminded me that we didn't actually speak until late Thursday afternoon, two days later. I called him with no regard to time to leave a message, but knowing your best friend in the world is alive and knowing that they're okay are very different things. New York's bubble of fuckery rendered cell phones spotty, inside and out. It wasn't until he could get to a phone in the teacher's breakroom that his call finally connected, and I could hear that the only thing more terrifying than living through it, was not knowing.

Lori.

Sporadic messages relayed between family and my partner's somehow-working phone mitigated the shock midday Tuesday, letting each other know we were both alive. Her getting back to Manhattan was like a zombified John Hughes movie. *No planes.* Renting a minivan, driving across never-before-empty Pennsylvania and Jersey turn-pikes, being rerouted around the city to a fucking Connecticut train station. Only to be dumped at the Bronx/Upper West Side border late at night. After two more trains, she finally returned to her version of the empty apartment, as I was finishing a shift I was never supposed to have.

Long after midnight, I walked the six blocks home to 81st and 2nd through already sprouting vigils. I couldn't wait any longer. Keys out, I ran up the four flights to defeat our double locks. The cylinders clicked and I opened our door.

Lori.

Wearing only my Mentor Fire Department T-shirt. Proudly like a dress. Waiting, with arms trembling. Waiting, with that beautiful face that only she can make. Scared and relieved and happy all at the same time. Tears bulging in the corners, but her smile too wide to let them out.

I dropped my bag and she kissed me.

Kissed me like stealing back seventy-five years of lost kisses.

Fuck, we were alive!

We sat with our legs locked on our too-tiny loveseat, our foreheads together. I cupped Lori's face. She held my hands. No words needed.

Not for hours.

Acknowledgements

Thank you, DSH, for reading an old pile of field notes and immediately being convinced that I had a much larger story to tell. For delivering on every promise and dealing with my impatience. For your great suggestions and supporting me as a customer, fan, and best of all, as a friend.

Thanks to Miette, for taking a chance on this complete unknown. For wishing books like mine into existence. For being able to say Whiskey Tit anytime I like!

Thanks to Dr. Sheryl Thompson. For your thoughtful introduction and thorough medical review. For being a shining example of what medicine should be. And for being a friend and inspiration long after we stopped working together.

Thanks to Aunt Nancy for inspiring a love of art and imagination that have made so much possible.

Thanks to everyone who has supported Collectible Science Fiction, without which my second life and the connections that made *American Triage* possible never would have happened.

Thanks to the Michael Rosenfeld Gallery for entrusting me with Nancy Grossman's art. It is a true privilege.

Thanks to Rock (aka Scott Peterson) for the Devil's 8 Ball and being the best friend anyone could ever hope to have.

Thanks to Mom for blueberry-peach cobbler and making me her sunshine. For being tough as hell. And for still taking care of people every day.

Thanks to Dad for Strat-O-Matic Baseball and surrounding me with books before I knew I loved them. For making Cleveland my hometown.

Thanks to my incredible daughters, Sammi and Syd. My most biased beta readers who clapped with each paragraph and who love their Dadoo no matter what.

And thanks to my amazing wife, Lori. My life's biggest fan. Whose support allowed me to leave 25 years in medicine behind with another 20 on the table. Whose sacrifice has made the entirety of our beautiful life together possible. And without whom, none of this would matter.

About the Author

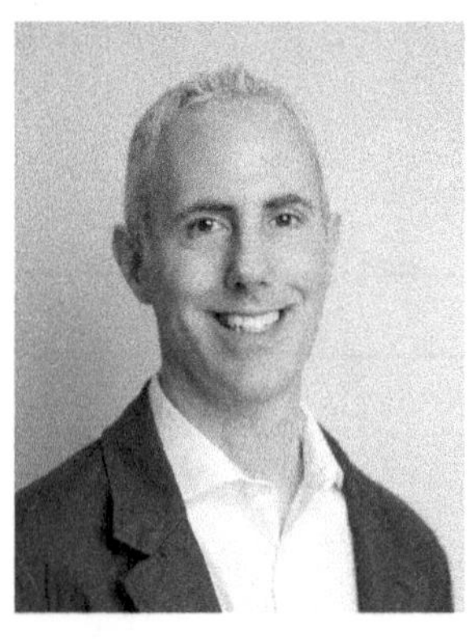

Adam Axler is a proud Clevelander. He has bartended at B-Dubs, worked as a firefighter/medic in Mentor, Ohio, and driven ambulances in New York from Yonkers to the World Trade Center. After almost two decades as a physician assistant, he has spent the last ten years as the happy owner of Collectible Science Fiction (collectiblesciencefiction.com), an online bookstore that makes many people happy as well. When not reading, collecting, or selling books, he enjoys his daily walks with his wife, Lori, and being the best girl-dad he can be to Sammi and Syd.

About the Artist

NANCY GROSSMAN (b.1940)

A master of sculpture, drawing, and collage, Nancy Grossman was born in New York City. She studied painting under Richard Lindner at Pratt Institute, earning her BFA degree in 1962.

In the late 1960s, Grossman began creating her famous leather-covered head sculptures along with her related collages and drawings. While their size, shape, and facial features suggest masculinity, she refers to them as self-portraits, implying the mutability of gender and demonstrating that all artwork offers something of the artist.

Grossman's work is represented in numerous museum collections worldwide including the Art Institute of Chicago (IL); Museum Boijmans Van Beuningen (Rotterdam, The Netherlands); Crystal Bridges Museum of American Art (AR); Israel Museum (Jerusalem); Los Angeles County Museum of Art (CA); The Menil Collection (Houston, TX); The Metropolitan Museum of Art; Museum of Modern Art (New York, NY); Nasher Sculpture Center (Dallas, TX); Smithsonian American Art Museum (Washington, DC); and the Whitney Museum of American Art (New York, NY).

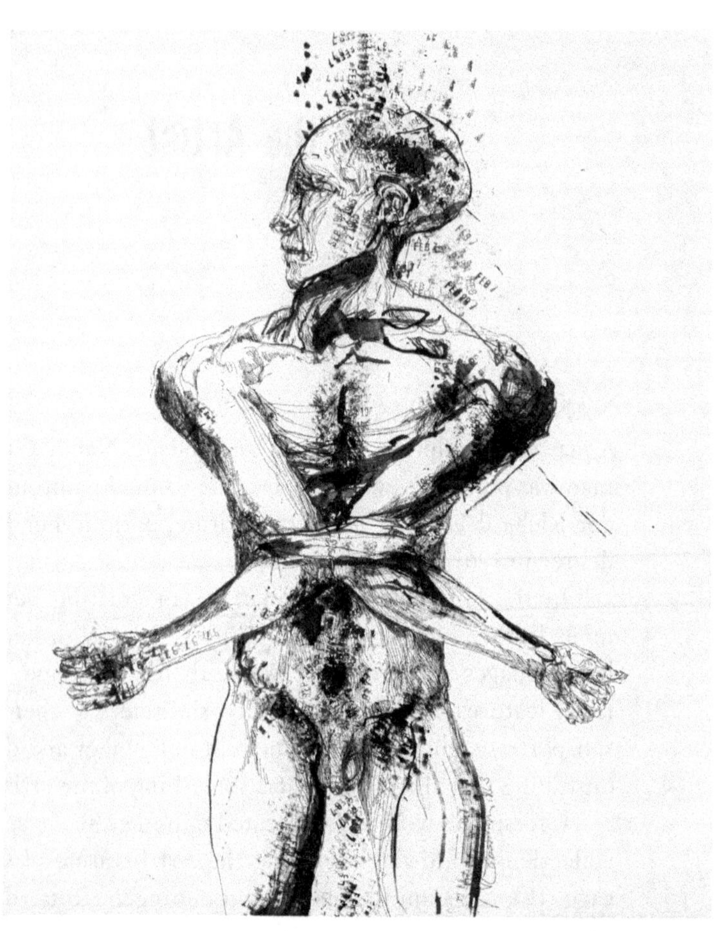

Nancy Grossman (b.1940), Male Figure Bound at Elbows with Head Turned Right Yet To Be Titled, 1963, ink on paper, 16 3/4 x 13 7/8 inches / 42.5 x 35.2 cm, signed; Collection of halley k harrisburg and Michael Rosenfeld, New York; © Nancy Grossman, Courtesy of Michael Rosenfeld Gallery LLC, New York, NY

American Triage

About the Publisher

Whisk(e)y Tit is committed to restoring degradation and degeneracy to the literary arts. We work with authors who are unwilling to sacrifice intellectual rigor, unrelenting playfulness, and visual beauty in our literary pursuits, often leading to texts that would otherwise be abandoned in today's largely homogenized literary landscape. In a world governed by idiocy, our commitment to these principles is an act of civil service and civil disobedience alike.